PRACTICAL OPHTHALMOLOGY

Also by James Y. Hung:

Finding Fat Lady's Shoe: A Memoir of Growing up in Hong Kong and Malaysia. (2013)

FOB in Paradise: A Memoir. (2014)

Silk Road on My Mind (2015)

Available through Amazon in paperback and Kindle e-book. E-book also available through Barnes & Noble.

Finding Fat Lady's Shoe

An intensely reflective tale of a family uprooted by war, cast adrift onto a sea of uncertainty.—Kirkus Review

Dr. James Hung's life story echoes others that will probably never be written, and offers a fascinating perspective on Hong Kong's recent past that deserves to be widely read. [4 stars out of 5]—South China Morning Post

FOB in Paradise

Hung has written an absorbing and witty book. Dramatic, nuanced vignettes and vivid descriptions of people and places create a rich tapestry that shows the medical profession at its best and worst. —Kirkus Review

Silk Road on My Mind

Hung is an endearing mix of benevolence, wryness, and curiosity.... there is an appealing Marco Polo–ishness to his project: a boundless wonder for a society unlike his own, not for its differences but for the infinitely recognizable humanity at its center.—Kirkus Review

PRACTICAL OPHTHALMOLOGY

A CONCISE MANUAL FOR THE NON-OPHTHALMOLOGIST

James Y. Hung, MD

Practical Ophthalmology: A Concise Manual for the Non-ophthalmologist

Copyright © 2016 by James Y. Hung.

ISBN: 0692748601
EAN: 978-0692748602 (James Y Hung)

Cover by Tony Ton
Editing and text design by Anne Correia

CONTENTS

PREFACE

Ophthalmology is so specialized that it essentially has its own language, which is not easy for health care workers outside of the specialty to understand. When I considered writing a book about ophthalmology, I first debated whether or not there was a need for another ophthalmology book, and concluded that one should be written solely with the non-ophthalmologists in mind.

The population is growing older in many countries and eye problems are more prevalent as we age; primary care providers must have a solid understanding of the more common eye disorders in order to serve these patients adequately.

During the past two decades, ophthalmology has undergone a great deal of change. Many eye surgeries are now done in outpatient centers, away from the hospital. Some eye departments have their own buildings, segregating the ophthalmologists from the rest of the medical community, widening the gap of communication. Many medical students graduate never having had a rotation in ophthalmology (I was one), as it is only an elective in most medical schools and not required.

This concise book can be read in a day or two. It will provide the reader with core knowledge on how to provide basic eye care and when to refer a patient elsewhere. Only conditions that are likely to be seen in the primary care setting are discussed.

In many developing countries, only a handful of ophthalmologists serve the entire population, which can number in the millions. It is hoped that this book would encourage primary care providers to offer basic eye care and help them work better with ophthalmologists and non-physician eye care providers (who, in some countries, have been trained to do eye surgeries).

The subject matter in the book varies widely from the supplies and equipment needed to provide basic eye care, to how to do an eye examination, basic optics, treatment of corneal problems, infections, glaucoma, and neurological and vascular diseases concerning the eye.

My foundation plans to distribute this book free of charge to as many health care providers in developing countries as possible. The book, as well as photos of clinical conditions, can be downloaded free of charge from my website: www.jamesyhungbooks.com.

I want to thank the American Academy of Ophthalmology for granting me permission to use a few of its drawings in the book.

James Y. Hung, MD, FACS
Honolulu, Hawaii 2016

AUTHOR'S NOTE

When I spent two weeks in Apia, Western Samoa at the General Hospital in 2014, working in the eye department, a young house officer was shadowing me. We saw a patient with a strange looking cyst in his retina, and the first thought that came to my mind was Toxocara canis—a parasitic infection spread by dog feces—as there were many feral dogs around the city. With both thumbs working away on his iPhone, Sala was able to get the information on Toxocara canis within two minutes, including an image almost identical to the retina finding in our patient. I was impressed. Most young doctors today are probably just as tech savvy as Sala.

My point is that ophthalmology is a visual specialty. We often make a diagnosis by having seen at least one such case before. Ideally, this book should have been printed in color, full of pictures of clinical conditions. Unfortunately, printing in color is five times as expensive as black and white, and concerns about accessibility and affordability took precedence.

I suggest the best way to use this book is to download photos from the Internet of the diseases and conditions described. The photos will likely be clearer—and more abundant, providing images of different stages and from various angles—than those printed on paper. Practically any clinical conditions can be found online; and YouTube also has videos of different eye surgeries, demonstrations of performing tests, and methods of examining the eye. This book should be used as a starting point to building the ophthalmology knowledge that a reader desires to acquire.

The smart phone now has several adapters for taking photos of the fundus. If you are uncertain of a diagnosis, such as whether or not a diabetic patient's retinopathy needs laser treatment, you can send the photos for consultation. Telemedicine has improved eye care tremendously, often saving patients and their families the time and money required for an in-person consultation.

I hope you find this book helpful in your practice.

Thank you.

James Y. Hung, MD, FACS

CHAPTER 1: EQUIPMENT & SUPPLIES

THE LEVEL OF EYE CARE YOU WISH TO PROVIDE TO YOUR PATIENTS DEPENDS ON YOUR COMFORT LEVEL AND TRAINING. If you are unsure of a diagnosis or course of treatment, never hesitate to refer your patient to an ophthalmologist.

BASIC EQUIPMENT

1. Ophthalmoscope
2. Hand flashlight
3. Binocular magnifying loupe
4. Visual acuity chart (Snellen)
5. The Rosenbaum pocket vision screener
6. Amsler grid
7. Schiotz tonometer
8. Smartphone as a retinal camera (optional)

Direct Ophthalmoscope

Eye examination was one of the more difficult skills I had to learn in medical school. We practiced looking into each other's eyes for hours, and still it wasn't easy. During my internship, family practice residency and ER days, trying look at the optic discs of older patients with small pupils and cataracts was truly challenging.

During my ophthalmology residency, I realized that ophthalmologists have an advantage over the primary care docs because they always dilate the pupils, and they have all kinds of equipment to help them look into their patients' eyes, including the indirect ophthalmoscope and special contact lenses with mirrors.

Now, for those of you who are tech savvy, there are several adapters that you can get for your smartphone to take photos of the fundus. Your office assistant can also be taught to do this. The photos can be compared to images of similar conditions; and they can also be sent to an ophthalmologist for advice on whether laser treatment would be indicated.

Binocular Loupe

If you practice in a rural area and the ophthalmologist is far away, you may have to remove a corneal foreign body. You will appreciate the binocular loupe, which provides you with depth perception.

Visual Acuity Chart

If you do physical examinations for employers, insurance, driver's licenses, etc., visual acuity is one of the items that you have to fill in on the forms. The Snellen chart (page 12) is easy to use and the exam can be done by your assistant.

Rosenbaum Pocket Vision Screener

If it is difficult or not possible to check visual acuity with the Snellen chart, such as with a bedridden or uncooperative patient, a Rosenbaum Pocket Vision Screener can be used. If the patient normally wears reading glasses, this test should be done with them on. It should be read one eye at a time at a distance of about 14 inches or 35 centimeters.

Amsler Grid

As the population gets older, the incidence of macular degeneration increases. Now with wonder drugs like Lucentis, a drug that will stop new vessels from doing more damage to the central vision, early detection is more important than ever. Amsler Grid testing can help with a diagnosis (pages 7-9).

Schiotz Tonometer

This is a mechanical device that you place on the cornea to measure the intraocular pressure. It's unlikely that you would be taking care of glaucoma patients, but if someone comes in with eye pain and you see no sign of infection and the cornea is intact—and the ophthalmologist is far away—you can easily check the pressure to rule out glaucoma, especially of the angle closure variety.

This tonometer (page 10) lasts forever and is easy to use. It costs around $200 in the US, and much less in some developing countries.

BASIC MEDICATIONS AND SUPPLIES

1. Topical anesthetics: proparacaine 0.5% or tetracaine 0.5%
2. Sterile fluorescein paper
3. Mydriatics: phenylephrine 2.5% and/or tropicamide (Mydriacyl) 1%
4. Miotics: pilocarpine 1%
5. Antibacterial Agents
6. Sterile solutions for irrigation
7. Eye pads
8. Eye shields
9. Sterile cotton-tipped applicators
10. Corticosteroid drops or ointment (or corticosteroid/antibiotic combination)

Topical Anesthetics

Proparacaine and tetracaine are most commonly used for topical anesthesia. They are said to have equivalent anesthetic potency. Anesthesia begins within 1 minute of application and lasts for 15 to 20 minutes. It numbs both the cornea and conjunctiva.

The cornea has extensive nerve endings and is one of the most sensitive organs in the body, making it ideal for topical anesthetics.

Fluorescein Paper

These come as single use sterile paper strips. The dye on the strips will detect corneal injury as well as locate foreign bodies.

Mydriatics

Dilating the pupil for fundus examination is worrisome for those who have never taken an ophthalmology rotation (like me). The primary concern is causing angle closure glaucoma in the patient. Of the tens of thousands of eyes dilated in my clinic, I cannot recall one patient who suffered that complication.

In one case, I carefully watched an elderly woman after dilation because of her narrow angle, and she did have a rise of her intraocular pressure and further narrowing of the angle. She was diagnosed with narrow angle with intermittent closure and was treated with one drop of 1% pilocarpine q.h.s. (4% pilocarpine may cause headache. The treatment of angle closure glaucoma is with laser iridotomy—a 15-minute procedure in the office.)

Tropicamide 1% (Mydriacyl) is the most commonly used drop for dilating the pupil. It takes 20 to 25 minutes for maximal dilation and the duration of the effect is 4 to 8 hours.

Phenylephrine 2.5% can also be used for dilation. The effect begins within 30 minutes and lasts 2 to 3 hours. Over the decades, several cases of elderly patients were reported to have suffered myocardial infarction that might be linked to the 10% phenylephrine, so it is now rarely used. Phenylephrine should not be used with known cardiac patients.

Antibacterial Agents

The drug I recommend for the primary care provider is sulfacetamide, which comes in 10% and 30% ophthalmic solution as well as 10% ophthalmic ointment. Sulfonamides are the most commonly used drugs for bacterial conjunctivitis because they are effective against both gram-positive and gram-negative organisms. It is very inexpensive and few people are allergic to it. Its use is not complicated by secondary fungal infection as can occur with some other antibiotics.

A bottle of drops or a tube of ointment of 10% sulfacetamide costs less than a dollar in many developing countries and is freely available without prescription.

Other antibiotics include tetracycline, erythromycin, aminoglycosides and fluoroquinolones. Ophthalmic ointment is much easier to use on a child than drops. Topical chloramphenicol is an extremely effective antibacterial, which is commonly used outside the US and is very inexpensive.

Irrigation Solutions

Any contact lens solution will do. If a patient has a chemical burn, the eye would need to be irrigated copiously. In case of emergency, any clean water can be used.

Eye Pads

If a patient has a corneal abrasion, a firm eye pad keeps the eye from moving under the lid. A corneal abrasion can be extremely painful, and bed rest and the eye pad will help keep the patient comfortable as well as speed up the healing process.

Eye Shield

If a patient has been hitting metal against metal and a piece of it is suspected to have entered the eye, a shield should be placed over the eye to prevent further damage. Immediate referral to an ophthalmologist is indicated.

Sterile Cotton-tipped Applicator

This is an item that every medical office should have. It can be used to remove a corneal foreign body as well as check the cornea for leaks if an injury is suspected. It also can be used to examine and explore the extent of injury to the conjunctiva and lid.

Caution for Corticosteroid and Topical Anesthetic Use

Topical corticosteroids are very effective for severe allergic conjunctivitis and ocular inflammation, but they also have severe adverse effects on the eye. They should never be used to treat herpes simplex, bacterial or fungal infections. They may lead to fungal keratitis following a corneal foreign body of vegetable matter, and can also cause posterior subcapsular cataract and secondary open-angle glaucoma.

Use corticosteroids to treat allergic conjunctivitis only when you are certain that it is allergic and not something else. Use only for a short period.

Never send a patient with a corneal injury home with a bottle of topical anesthetic. If used inappropriately, it can lead to severe complications such as corneal ulcer and even blindness.

OTHER MEDICATIONS
Diamox (Acetazolamide) 500mg tablets
Glycerin
Injectable anesthetic with epinephrine 1:10,000

THE AMSLER GRID

With this test anyone can check their central vision at home. A patient should use the Amsler grid to test the central vision every day to detect any changes that may be caused by worsening age-related macular degeneration (AMD) or other macular disorders.

Follow these steps while looking at the grid on the following page:

1. If you usually wear reading glasses, put them on.
2. Hold the grid at a normal reading distance, about 12-14 inches away from your face.
3. Using only your right eye (left eye closed), look at the dot in the center of the grid. Make sure that you can see the entire grid.
4. If any of the lines in the grid look distorted, blurry, or missing, write down what you see.
5. Repeat these steps with your left eye while your right eye is closed. If any of these changes are new, call your retina doctor the same day.

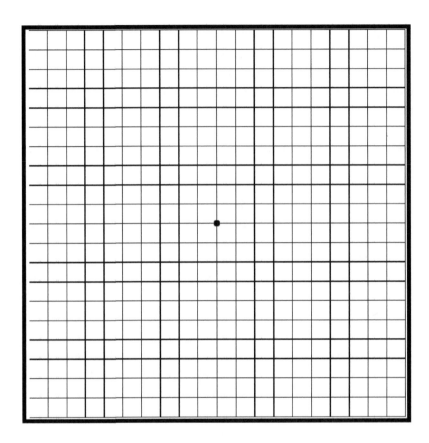

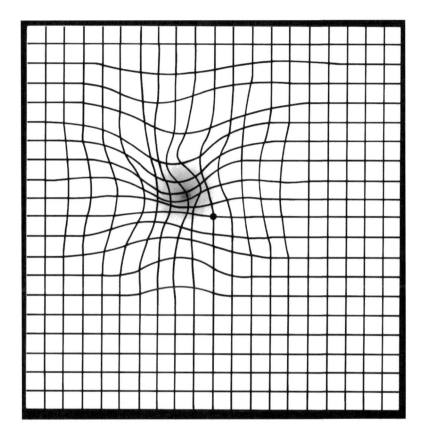

If the patient sees the lines as wavy, seeming to bend or appearing gray, fuzzy or missing in certain areas of the grid (one example is shown above), this indicates that some damage has been done to the macula, and the patient should be referred to a retinal specialist for further evaluation.

TECHNIQUE OF SCHIOTZ TONOMETRY

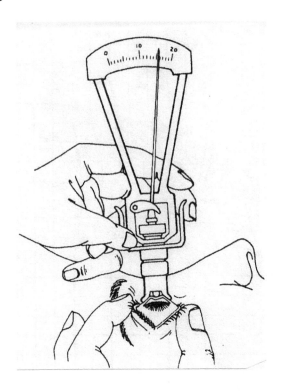

Anesthetize the cornea with topical proparacaine or tetracaine.

Ask the patient to lie in a supine position looking directly upward, fixing on a spot in the ceiling.

Separate the lids to keep them from touching the eyeball, taking care not to put any pressure on the eye.

Place the tonometer gently in a vertical position over the cornea with the plunger exerting its full weight.

The pointer will give a steady reading within 0.5 mm in either direction.

Keep the part of the tonometer that touches the cornea sterile.

IPHONE WITH ATTACHMENT FOR FUNDUS PHOTOGRAPH

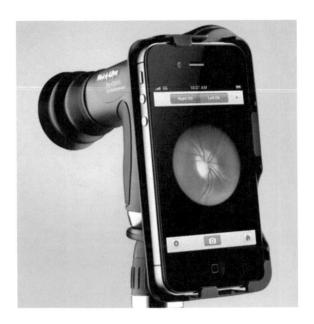

There are several models on the market that are compatible with other smartphones. (Search Google for, "iPhone, smartphone for fundus photography" and you will find the different options.)

An assistant can be trained to do this job.

This is especially useful for diabetic patients. The photos can be compared for possible progression of the retinopathy.

The photos can be stored in the EMR system or can be sent to a colleague for consultation, especially if the patient is elderly and lives far away from an ophthalmologist.

SNELLEN CHART

$\frac{20}{200}$	**E**	200 FT / 61 M	1
$\frac{20}{100}$	**F P**	100 FT / 30.5 M	2
$\frac{20}{70}$	**T O Z**	70 FT / 21.3 M	3
$\frac{20}{50}$	**L P E D**	50 FT / 15.2 M	4
$\frac{20}{40}$	**P E C F D**	40 FT / 12.2 M	5
$\frac{20}{30}$	**E D F C Z P**	30 FT / 9.14 M	6
$\frac{20}{25}$	**F E L O P Z D**	25 FT / 7.62 M	7
$\frac{20}{20}$	**D E F P O T E C**	20 FT / 6.10 M	8
$\frac{20}{15}$	L E F O D P C T	15 FT / 4.57 M	9
$\frac{20}{13}$	F D P L T C E O	13 FT / 3.96 M	10
$\frac{20}{10}$	F E C O L C F T D	10 FT / 3.05	11

NEAR VISION CARD

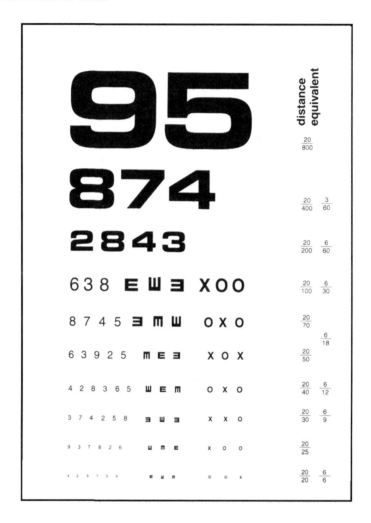

This card is used to measure near visual acuity. Although it is close to the correct size, a true-to-scale copy can be printed from the Internet. The card is held in good light 40 cm (16 inches) from the eye. Record vision for each eye separately with and without glasses. Presbyopic patients should read through bifocal segment. Check myopes with glasses only.

CHAPTER 2: HISTORY AND EXAMINATION

As this book has been written mainly for primary care practitioners, it is assumed that examinations will be done without the benefit of a slit lamp, using a magnifying glass or loupe.

We all know how important a good history and examination are in the care of a patient. When a patient shows up in a non-ophthalmologist's office with an eye problem, the practitioner has to be selective and realize that he or she is not providing vision care or complete eye care, but just addressing the eye problem for that visit.

HISTORY

The history no doubt relates to the reason the patient is in the office, such as red eye, eye pain or discomfort, a foreign body in the eye, seeing double, seeing floaters and so on. The practitioner needs to know how long this condition has been going on, if it is getting worse, better or remains unchanged, and other things that might be related to the presenting problem. The practitioner should be as accurate and precise as possible.

A history of eye injuries and the use of eye drops such as corticosteroid would be pertinent information to gather when dealing with most eye problems. It can also be useful to learn if any herbs have been taken orally or applied topically.

THE OCULAR EXAMINATION
(selective and relevant pertaining to each visit)

Hands and fingernails should be clean, and after each patient, especially those with infections, the hands should be washed.

Try to develop the habit of always examining the right eye first and the left eye second, even if the patient only complains of a problem in the left eye. This routine ensures that the eye with the problem can be compared to the "healthy" eye.

Visual acuity measurement should usually be done with any patient who comes to a primary care provider's office with an eye problem.

Cross-confrontation visual field testing may need to be done if the patient is running into things or experiencing other visual perception problems.

Eye movement may be tested to evaluate the integrity of the extra-ocular muscles.

Examination of the eyelids, sclera, cornea and conjunctiva may be needed.

Pupillary reactivity and size may be recorded if relevant.

The anterior chamber may be examined.

Check for opacity of the lens or vitreous if needed.

Examination of the macula, optic nerve and retina may be done.

Measurement of the intraocular pressure may be done.

As the comfort levels of primary care practitioners varies so much, I recommend that common sense be used as to how much examination is needed for a particular visit. In the case of a patient with a red eye, which could be contagious, the longer he or she is kept in the office, the greater the chances of the infection spreading to the staff and other patients. My philosophy is when a patient comes in with an eye infection, see him or her as soon as possible, prescribe the appropriate medication, and don't keep him or her around to spread the infection.

A useful acuity test is the **pinhole (PH) test**. The pinhole test is performed on a patient with diminished visual acuity, to determine whether it is due to a refractive error or from an organic disease such as macular degeneration. If you don't have a pinhole occluder, you can create one by making several pinholes, 0.5–2 mm in diameter, in a card. The patient looks through one of the holes one eye at a time without wearing corrective lenses. If the visual acuity is improved by looking through the pinholes, the problem is refractive. If not, it is organic. The pinhole effect works by blocking peripheral light waves, which are most distorted by refractive error.

Many primary care offices have assistants who can do the **Snellen chart test** (page 12), which consists of letters or numbers printed in decreasing sizes according to an international standard. In the US, the distance at which a patient reads the chart is measured in feet, i.e. 20/20; and in the EU, it is measured in meters, as in 6/6. If the examination room is less than 20 feet long, then use a distance of ten feet and make the adjustment accordingly. If a person can see the 20/40 line at 20 feet, then he or she should be able to see the 20/20 line at 10 feet, and so on.

If the patient's vision is so poor that the figures on the chart cannot be read, direct the patient's attention to the outstretched fingers on your hand and ask the patient to count the number of fingers you are holding up at various distances, such as at 2 feet, 4 feet, etc. Record the distance of the best finger-counting vision.

If the patient cannot count fingers even at close range, then the light projection test may be used. Test the patient to determine if focal light from a flashlight can be seen in each of the four retinal quadrants by holding the light about 4 inches from the eye in front of the face and pointing in toward the eye. Ask the patient to point to the direction of the light. If the patient is correct in in all four quadrants, record the results as "accurate light projection." If the patient makes a mistake in one or more quadrants, then record it as "inaccurate light projection." This test is useful if the patient is being screened for possible cataract surgery. If the patient has accurate light projection, cataract surgery would most likely benefit the patient. If the patient has inaccurate light projection, it may mean a problem in the retina. If the patient has NLP (no light perception), cataract surgery may not benefit this patient and further testing should be done. Even for a patient with extremely dense cataracts, some light usually passes through.

Common abbreviations used for recording visual acuity:
- V (vision)
- RE (right eye) or OD (oculus dexter)
- LE (left eye) or OS (oculus sinister)
- NV (near vision)
- PH (pinhole)
- CF (counting fingers): example, CF at 2 ft., 4ft., etc.
- NLP (no light perception)

Red Reflex

The red reflex tests the light reflected from the blood vessels of the choroid. With a +5 diopter lens in the aperture of the ophthalmoscope, at a distance of about 8 inches from the cornea, check to see if the pupil appears red, and is identical in both eyes. A good red reflex means that everything along the visual axis is clear. Any media opacity, i.e., cornea, lens or vitreous, will interrupt the red reflex and give abnormal results.

Examination of the Retina

After examining for media opacities, move slowly closer to the patient's eye while dialing in smaller plus (+) lens numbers until the ophthalmoscope is a few centimeters from the eye. Adjust the distance until the retina becomes clear. Then examine the optic nerve head (optic disc) first, followed by the small arteries and veins. Then examine the macula by asking the patient to look directly at the light.

Use of the handheld ophthalmoscope to examine the inside of the eye through an un-dilated pupil is not easy and requires practice. Keep working with it and eventually it will become more routine.

DIRECT OPHTHALMOSCOPE

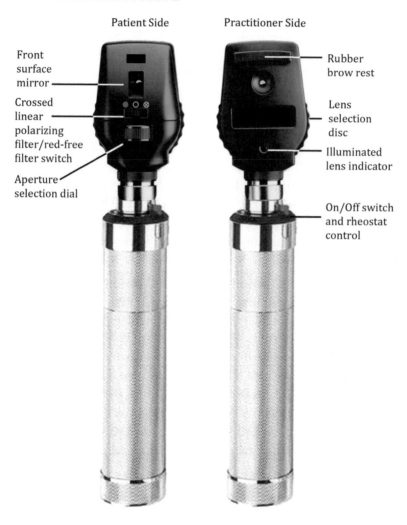

Patient Side   Practitioner Side

Front surface mirror

Crossed linear polarizing filter/red-free filter switch

Aperture selection dial

Rubber brow rest

Lens selection disc

Illuminated lens indicator

On/Off switch and rheostat control

There are different models of direct ophthalmoscope. The newer ones have some functions that are seldom needed, many of which you can ignore.

The black numbers on the lens selection disc represent plus lenses—to correct hyperopia.

The red numbers represent minus lenses—to correct myopia.

The smaller white round beam is for small pupils.

The larger round beam is most frequently used and provides the largest view of the fundus, but it is only good for a large pupil, i.e., usually dilated.

Most of the other beam shapes are seldom used.

Be familiar with all the functions of the ophthalmoscope.

APERTURES (viewing holes):

Small Aperture: Provides easy view of the fundus through an undilated pupil. Always start the examination with this aperture and proceed to micro aperture if pupil is particularly small and/or sensitive to light.

Large Aperture: Standard aperture for dilated pupil and general examination of the eye.

Micro Spot Aperture: Allows easy entry into very small, undilated pupils.

Slit Aperture: Helpful in determining various elevations of lesions, particularly tumors and edematous discs.

PROPER WAY TO HOLD AN OPHTHALMOSCOPE

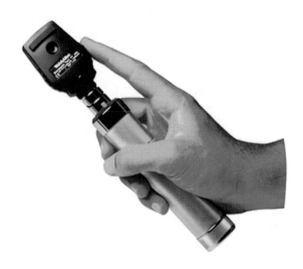

The index finger turns the lens selection disc to locate the lens that focuses the image most clearly.

Red-Free Filter: Excludes red rays from examination field for easy identification of veins, arteries, and nerve fibers.

Some people find it confusing to think about their own glasses and the patients' glasses. The way to do it is to set all the numbers on the ophthalmoscope to "0". Have the patient remove his or her glasses. You can wear your own or remove them. Contact lenses can stay in.

The room should be dim but not too dark. Explain to the patient what you are going to do and that the bright light can temporarily dazzle them.

Position the patient so that he or she is comfortable but sitting up—if possible.

If you decide to dilate, put one drop of 1% tropicamide (Mydriacil) in each eye and wait 15 to 30 minutes. Maximal dilation can be obtained by using Mydriacil and Neo-Synephrine simultaneously.

Even with dilation, only about a third of the fundus is visible. The area most visible is the posterior pole (including the disc and the macula). You should be able to see the ocular findings of many systemic diseases such as diabetes and hypertension.

Your patient should fixate on a specific target such as a piece of paper with a big "X" on the wall. This is important so that the patient does not move his or her eyes.

Examine the patient's right eye with your right eye and vice versa. Try to keep your other eye open, which may not be easy and takes practice. If you can't, do whatever you are comfortable with.

Begin at arm's length by shining the ophthalmoscope light into the patient's pupil; you will see the red-reflex (the pupil appears red instead of black when the ophthalmoscope is not used). *Media opacities (corneal scar, cataract, vitreous hemorrhage and asteroid hyalosis) obscure the red reflex.*

Rest your hand on the patient's forehead and use your thumb to hold his or her lid open. Follow the red reflex until your forehead rests on your thumb–you should see the optic disc. If it is out of focus, without moving your head, turn the lens selection disc either way. If the disc becomes clearer, keep turning. If it becomes blurrier, turn the dial the other way. It is difficult to see more than one disc diameter with the visual field of a direct ophthalmoscope. You have to tilt the instrument simultaneously with your head to different positions to have a composite picture of the fundus.

Look for the optic disc size, color, cup disc ratio, margins, hemorrhages, new vessels and collaterals. Pale and clearly demarcated disc indicate optic atrophy. New vessels on the disc suggest proliferative diabetic retinopathy (there are other causes of new vessels). Yellow-gray disc with blurred margins with or without hemorrhages suggests papilledema.

Look for venous pulsation. If it is present, it strongly suggests that there is no papilledema, because venous pulsation is one of the first things to disappear with papilledema. The absence of venous pulsation does not mean much since it may be difficult to detect in normal people.

From the disc, follow the vessels to look for arteriosclerotic and hypertensive changes. Look as far as the mid-peripheral for hemorrhages, exudates, scars and pigmented lesions. Examine the arteries and veins (slightly thicker); the A/V ratio is about 3/5. Check the arterioles for normal light reflex. Look for copper or silver wiring—a sign of thickening of the arteriolar media found in eyes with long standing hypertension. Examine the area adjacent to these vessels for micro-aneurysms, exudates, venous beading, venous loops and abnormal new vessels.

To examine the macula, have the patient look into your light. The foveal reflex is seen better with a green (red-free) filter and is two disc diameters away from the disc and 1.5 degrees below the horizontal. Look for hard exudates, hemorrhages and pigmentary changes in the macula.

I will again discuss dilation of the eye later. In the US, 1 in 1000 of the population over 40 will develop angle closure glaucoma. It is very unlikely that by dilating your patients' eyes, you will trigger an attack of angle closure. If that should happen, the symptoms are obvious and easily treated (see chapter on glaucoma).

INDIRECT OPHTHALMOSCOPY

This is a technique used by ophthalmologists involving a head-mounted, prism-directed light source coupled with the use of a condensing lens, usually +20 or +28. The image is real and inverted, as well as stereoscopic, covering ten times the area of a direct ophthalmoscope. It has many advantages over the direct, but the learning curve is steep and the equipment is expensive and cumbersome; and, in addition, the eye is usually viewed through a dilated pupil.

PROPER TECHNIQUE TO INSTILL EYE DROPS

1. Wash your hands.
2. Have the patient seated, with the head tilted back, eyes looking up.
3. Pull the lower lid down gently to expose the palpebral conjunctiva.
4. Instill the drop(s) into the lower conjunctival fornix but not on the cornea directly. Do not touch the tip of the applicator or allow it to touch the patient's cornea.
5. Have the patient close both eyes for a few seconds.
6. Go over the above steps with the patient. If necessary, the technique may be modified to suit the patient.

CHAPTER 3: ANATOMY

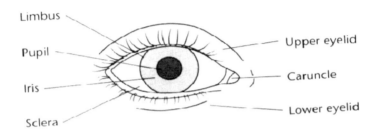

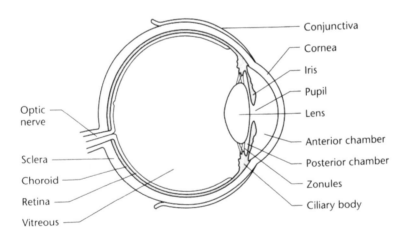

Cornea: The clear circular part of the front of the eyeball. It serves as a refractive surface (making light change direction) to help focus the object on the retina. It is avascular and gets its nutrients from the aqueous.

Pupil: The round opening in the center of the iris that controls the amount of light entering the eye.

Iris: The colored part of the eye that determines the size of the pupil. It is controlled by two muscles:

The sphincter muscle is responsible for closing the pupil in bright light and is innervated by the parasympathetic system. When a parasympathomimetic drug like Pilocarpine is instilled on the eye, it will cause the sphincter around the pupil to contract, making it small.

The other muscle in the iris, the radial or iris dilator muscle, runs from the edge of the pupil to its base and is innervated by the sympathetic system. When Phenylephrine, a sympathomimetic drug, is instilled on the eye, it causes this muscle to contract, thus pulling the pupil open.

Anterior chamber: The space between the cornea and the iris, which is filled with aqueous humor.

Posterior chamber: The small space filled with aqueous humor behind the iris and the front of the lens.

Conjunctiva: The almost transparent vascular mucous membrane covering the sclera (bulbar conjunctiva) and the inner surface of the eyelids (palpebral conjunctiva).

Lens: The biconvex clear structure behind the iris and pupil responsible for focusing the image on the retina.

Aqueous humor: The clear fluid that fills the space between the cornea and iris (anterior chamber) that nourishes the lens and cornea and gives the eye its shape.

Ciliary body: The structure that produces the aqueous humor. It also connects the lens—via suspensory ligaments—to the choroid. It contains the ciliary muscles, and when it contracts, it reduces the tension on the lens, making it more convex and focusing light closer to the lens, i.e., accommodation.

Suspensory ligaments: Ligaments between the lens and ciliary muscles.

Sclera: The thick white outer coat of the eye that is covered by the conjunctiva.

Choroid: The middle layer of the eye wall. It is vascular and pigmented. It provides blood supply to the outer retinal layers.

Retina: The innermost wall of the eye consisting of neural tissue. It sends visual signals to the brain via the optic nerve to be interpreted.

Macula: The area of the retina adjacent to the optic nerve that is responsible for central, fine vision.

Fovea: The center of the macula responsible for the finest vision.

Blind spot: The area where the optic nerve enters the eye and passes through the optic disc where there is no retina, hence the eye does not see anything at that spot.

Optic disc: Also called the optic nerve head. The usually yellow, circular junction, nasal to the macula, where the ganglion cell axons exit the eye, pick up a myelin sheath, and become the optic nerve. The optic nerve connects the eye to the brain.

Vitreous humor: A transparent, jelly-like substance that fills the eye behind the lens, extending to the retina and measuring about 4.5 cc in volume.

Uvea: The pigmented, vascular middle layer of the eye consisting of the choroid, ciliary body and iris.

CHAPTER 4: BASIC OPTICS

MYOPIA AND HYPEROPIA

An **emmetropic eyeball** is one with no refractive error. The absolute size of the eyeball is immaterial as long as it is the right length to go along with the other components of eye refraction, i.e., corneal curvature and lens power.

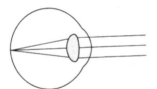

With an emmetropic eye, vision is considered "normal" and does not require corrective lenses. The image focuses directly onto the retina.

Myopia

Myopia is also called near-sightedness because myopes have good near vision but poor distant vision. The eyeball is too long for the refractive power of the cornea and lens. In general, we tend to associate a large eye with myopia. It is corrected with concave (minus) lenses. The concave lens brings the image into focus in front of the retina.

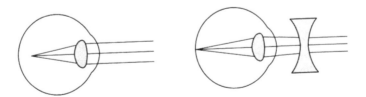

A myopic eye (left). The image forms too far in front of the retina. The concave lens (right) lengthens the focal point of the image to focus on the retina.

High myopia is diagnosed when the lens required to correct the near-sightedness is greater than 6 diopters. The elongation of the eyeball can be progressive throughout life, leading to degeneration of the retina. There is a higher incidence of retinal detachment in high myopes.

LASIK (Excimer laser in situ keratomileusis) for correction of myopia

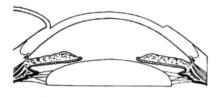

1. Corneal flap opened.

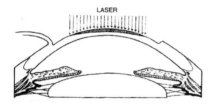

2. Ablation of stromal bed. Tissue removed (gray area).

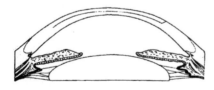

3. Flap replaced. Central cornea is now flatter (less myopic).

Hyperopia

Hyperopia or far-sightedness is corrected with convex (plus) lenses. It is called far-sightedness because one can see well at a distance but the near vision is poor. The eyeball is too short for the cornea and the power of the lens.

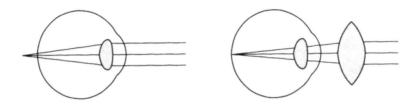

In a hyperopic eyeball (left), the focal point is located behind the retina. A convex lens (right) is required to accommodate.

For hyperopes, symptoms of eyestrain tend to have an earlier onset than myopes, and they often need reading glasses earlier than myopes because of the loss of accommodation. Because of the smaller eyeball, primary angle-closure glaucoma is more common in people with hyperopia, something often seen in East Asians, especially among the Chinese.

Presbyopia occurs when the lens loses its accommodation well enough to focus on near images as a result of age-related processes, rather than the anatomical factors that cause near- or far-sightedness. This occurs earlier (around age forty) in people with hyperopia and later in myopic eyes.

Bifocal glasses may be needed for people who need correction for both distant and near vision.

Reading glasses with power from +1.00 to +3.00 can be purchased in most drug stores. Suggest that your patients try them out and find the one (or ones) that meet their needs. Using drug store reading glasses will not damage the eyes.

APHAKIA

Aphakia refers to an eye that no longer has its own natural lens, usually following cataract surgery. A generation ago, many of the patients in developing countries who had cataract surgery were fitted with thick glasses to replace the optical power of the lens removed. The problem with such a correction is that the image the patient sees is about 30% larger than that of the lens inside the eye. This is a big concern for patients who are active, because the magnification of vision can cause them to misjudge their steps, resulting in falls.

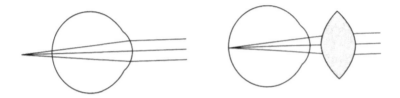

Image is 30% larger in aphakic patients corrected with spectacles.

Vision in an aphakic eye without correction is extremely blurry and the patient is usually considered essentially blind.

Pseudophakia is the term used to describe an eye with an intra-ocular lens (IOL). The quality of the intra-ocular lens has improved greatly over the last twenty years, and their price has reduced drastically. Now most patients even in the poorest countries receive an IOL following cataract surgery. The IOL usually corrects distant vision, but the patient still has to wear reading glasses. However, there are now all sorts of new IOLs, some of which enable the patient to see clearly at distance as well as near.

ASTIGMATISM

Astigmatism occurs when the cornea is not symmetrically round. Instead of being like a basketball, it is shaped like a football, with one meridian more curved than the meridian perpendicular to it. Imagine the front of the eye as the face of a clock. The line from 12 to 6 is the 90-degree meridian and from

3 to 9 is the 180-degree. The steepest and flattest meridians are called the principal meridians and are always 90 degree from each other. The irregular shape of the cornea in astigmatism patients causes light to focus on multiple points (either behind or in front of the retina, or both) instead of a single focus point, and the result is blurry or distorted vision. Eyestrain, squinting and headaches can also be symptoms of astigmatism.

Correction for regular astigmatism can usually be incorporated into eyeglasses. Refractive surgery can also sometimes be used to correct regular astigmatism.

Irregular astigmatism is far less common and is usually caused by diseases such as keratoconus, or by scarring after an eye injury. It is usually treated with rigid gas permeable contact lenses instead of corrective lenses.

Types of Astigmatism

Hyperopic astigmatism. One or both principal meridians are far-sighted, i.e., at least one focal point is located behind the retina. The image on the left is simple hyperopic and the one on the right is compound hyperopic. The short lines in the following diagrams indicate points of focus.

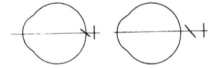

Mixed astigmatism. One principal meridian is near-sighted, and the other is far-sighted.

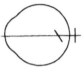

Myopic astigmatism. One or both meridians of the eye are near-sighted. The one on the left is compound myopic and the one on the right is simple myopic.

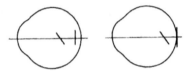

This is an example of simple myopic astigmatism:

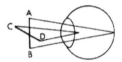

The vertical (90 degree) beam (AB) is focused on the retina and needs no correction.

The horizontal (180 degree) beam (CD) is focused anterior to the retina like that in a myopic eye.

The horizontal beam (CD) can be corrected with a myopic cylindrical lens.

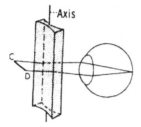

CONTACT LENSES

Contact lenses rest on the cornea. They have some advantages over regular glasses.

- They are often cosmetically more desirable.
- In patients with very high refractive error such as a plus 10, strong convex lenses are needed. This hyperopic patient's glasses would be very thick and the environment would appear magnified. The field of vision is also restricted with pronounced distortion when the patient looks through the edges of the glasses. The patient's eyes also appear magnified to the observer. A patient with high myopia sees the environment as smaller than normal and also experiences distortion when looking through the edge of the glasses. Their eyes appear small to the observer. A contact lens eliminates these problems.
- The vision of a patient with irregular astigmatism can be corrected with contact lenses.

The negative aspects of contact lenses are:

- Many people find them difficult to wear or hard to handle.
- If not worn properly, the eye can be damaged.
- They are generally more expensive than glasses.
- The contact lens wearer must live in a clean environment, which is not always possible in some developing countries.

There are many types of contact lenses and they continue to improve. It is a specialty in itself.

CHAPTER 5: EYELIDS, CONJUNCTIVA, CORNEA AND SCLERA

COMMON EYELID CONDITIONS

Blepharitis

Blepharitis is a common inflammation of the eyelids. It usually involves the lashes, lid margin and the meibomian glands (oil glands lining the lid margin that prevent drying of the eye's tear film). It is a frustrating condition for the patient as it can be very uncomfortable and include irritation, redness and tearing. It is also frustrating for the physician because it is a recurring condition, and patients often fail to understand why it cannot be cured.

In **anterior blepharitis**, the meibomian glands are not primarily involved. It occurs along the outside edge of the eyelid where the eyelashes attach, and symptoms can include irritation, itching, crusting along the lid or missing eyelashes.

In **posterior blepharitis**, the meibomian glands are inflamed, leading to blockage and cyst formation. It occurs along the inner edge of the eyelid where it touches the eyeball, and can also cause crusting, irritation and missing eyelashes.

Therapy is essentially life-long as it recurs frequently if meticulous lid hygiene is not followed. Lid hygiene involves scrubbing the eyelids with baby shampoo followed by warm compresses several times a day. Topical antibiotic drops and/or ointment may be needed. If the inflammation is severe, corticosteroid drops or ointment may be required. A combination of corticosteroid and antibiotic drops or ointment is often used.

In severe cases—when the condition recurs and there is excessive redness and irritation—in addition to the lid hygiene and topical treatment, oral doxycycline or minocycline 100 mg q.d. for 3 weeks may be prescribed. Longer courses may be needed in persistent cases. For pregnant women and children under 10, erythromycin 250 mg p.o. q.d may be substituted. Usually, when blepharitis becomes severe, the patient should see an ophthalmologist.

Hordeolum

A Hordeolum (or stye) is an acute infection involving the eyelash follicles (**external hordeolum**) or meibomian glands (**internal hordeolum**) and is commonly caused by Staphylococcus. It is usually painful and includes purulent discharge (pus). Treatment is the same as for blepharitis.

Chalazion

Chalazion is a chronic infection of a meibomian gland, which may be the result of a chronic hordeolum. It is usually not painful for the patient. Initial treatment is the same as for blepharitis. If the lesion does not resolve in a couple of weeks, incision and curettage from the inside of the lid through the conjunctiva may be needed.

CONJUNCTIVA

Red Eye

Red Eye or conjunctivitis is one of the most common conditions seen in the office. It is a general term that actually covers many different conditions. It is important to make the correct diagnosis before appropriate treatments can be initiated.

Conjunctivitis can be described as purulent or non-purulent.

Bacterial Conjunctivitis

Bacterial conjunctivitis is usually characterized by pus (purulent) discharge. It can be bilateral or unilateral. No enlarged pre-auricular lymph nodes are usually found.

The most common cause of mild conjunctivitis and blepharitis is Staphylococcus aureus. Most mild conjunctivitis can be treated with topical antibiotic drops and/or ointment. Any of the following antibiotics can be used for mild conjunctivitis: sulfacetamide, erythroymycin, bacitracin, tetracycline and others.

If the infection is severe, culture for identification of the bacteria should be done. Infection by Pseudomonas and Klebsiella can cause severe corneal destruction and can lead to blindness. If either of these bacterium are present in the culture, the patient should be treated by an ophthalmologist.

Viral Conjunctivitis

Viral conjunctivitis is non-purulent and can be caused by a number of viruses. It is usually bilateral and enlarged pre-auricular nodes are present. The conjunctiva is diffusely red because of the vascular reaction, and it may have watery discharge.

The infection may be spread by coughing or sneezing. A mask must be worn when examining this group of patients. The infection usually clears in a week to ten days. If the infection appears to be severe, an antibiotic drop or ointment such as tetracycline 1% twice a day for five days may be used to prevent secondary infection.

Epidemic Hemorrhagic Conjunctivitis

Epidemic hemorrhagic conjunctivitis or adenoviral conjunctivitis (pink eye) is an extremely contagious viral infection. It is usually bilateral and enlarged lymph nodes are typically not found. The cornea is usually not affected. The patient looks terrible because of the diffuse sub-conjunctival hemorrhage.

Mask and gloves must be worn when examining a patient with this infection. If there is an epidemic, such patients should be discouraged from coming to the office, as they can spread the disease further.

Tetracycline 1% ointment twice a day for seven days may be used to prevent secondary bacterial infection.

Allergic Conjunctivitis

Allergic conjunctivitis is non-purulent and may be seasonal. The primary symptom is itching, and the patient may give a history of "hay fever" and bronchial asthma. Visual acuity is usually not affected, and enlarged pre-auricular lymph nodes are not present. Careful examination of the bulbar (covering the eye) and tarsal (the fibrous connective tissue that supports the edge of the eyelid) conjunctiva may show papillae (small bumps) of vascular reaction.

Topical corticosteroid is the treatment in the acute phase, but the diagnosis must be correct before such treatment is started. Long-term use of topical corticosteroid use can cause cataract and secondary glaucoma.

Patients with chronic allergic conjunctivitis may use an antihistamine or non-steroidal drops to prevent recurrence. Zaditor (ketotifen) is now available as an OTC eye drop. It acts as a mast-cell stabilizer and antihistamine and is very effective.

Combination of pheniramine and naphazoline drops (OTC) can provide relief of itching and redness associated with seasonal allergic conjunctivitis.

Patients should be warned against over-use of ocular decongestants (usually a weak adrenergic stimulating drug such as phenylephrine hydrochloride 0.12%), which can result in rebound vasodilation of conjunctival vessels.

Subconjunctival Hemorrhage

This is a deep red hemorrhage under the conjunctiva, which can appear spontaneously or as a result of coughing, sneezing or straining. In the absence of trauma or adenoviral conjunctivitis (pink eye), no treatment is necessary. The patient should be reassured that the blood will clear in 2 to 3 weeks.

If the condition is frequent and recurrent, a medical workup may be necessary to rule out hypertension or a bleeding disorder.

CORNEA

Corneal foreign bodies are among the most common eye injuries. They should be addressed as soon as possible to prevent permanent damage. The foreign body could be anything: sand, a metal fragment, vegetable matter, etc.

A corneal foreign body usually causes pain and interferes with the vision. Topical anesthetic and sometimes fluorescein dye may be applied before performing the examination under a bright light with a loupe. Lid eversion may be necessary to expose a foreign body embedded in the tarsus of the upper lid.

A cotton-tipped applicator should be tried first, and if the foreign body cannot be removed with the cotton-tipped applicator, a 25-gauge needle with the bevel up can be tried next.

If the foreign body is a metal fragment that has been on the cornea for a few days and a rust ring has formed, the patient may need to be referred to an ophthalmologist for removal of the rust ring. A rust ring may cause scarring; and if it is in the visual axis, it may interfere with the vision. If it is in the peripheral cornea, and referral to an ophthalmologist is not possible, the rust ring may be left alone. A primary care physician comfortable at the slit lamp may be able to use a battery operated handheld burr (e.g., the Alger Brush Corneal Rust Ring Remover) to remove the rust ring.

An antibiotic ointment without corticosteroid should be instilled in the inferior fornix (the space in the fold of the lower lid) followed by an occlusive eye patch. The patient should be re-examined in 24 hours to confirm epithelial healing. A non-healing epithelial defect can lead to a corneal ulcer. These patients must see an ophthalmologist because the defect can be blinding.

Corneal Chemical Injuries

A corneal chemical injury is an emergency. Copious amount of clean water should be used to irrigate the eye(s). A drop of topical anesthetic may be necessary to help the patient keep the eye(s) open while being irrigated. If a tap is available, the patient's head should be placed under running water with the eye(s) open for at least five minutes. Examination with fluorescein dye is then done to evaluate the extent of the injury.

The worst injuries are caused by alkaline (basic) chemicals with a pH of greater than 7.0, which include many cleaning fluids and lye (sodium hydroxide compounds). These chemicals can penetrate the cornea in seconds. Irrigation of the eye should continue until the pH (tested with a litmus paper) becomes neutral.

Ultraviolet (UV) Burns

Welding arcs and sun lamps are the most common causes of light-induced injury to the cornea. These can be prevented by wearing UV-blocking plastic spectacles or shields when exposed to the rays. An eye with a UV burn may show edema on the lid, conjunctival hyperemia, and corneal punctate roughening of the epithelium.

The patient may come in with severe pain, photophobia and spasm of the lid.

Treatment is a short-acting cycloplegic drop such as cyclopentolate 1% to relieve ciliary spasm, and topical antibiotic ointment. A semi-pressure dressing with the eyes well closed underneath should be applied and left on for 24 hours. A patient in severe pain may need analgesics and sedatives. The burn will usually heal within 24 to 48 hours.

Hyphema

Hyphema or blood in the anterior chamber is usually caused by a severe contusion to the eyeball, such as being hit in the eye by a baseball. It is treated with bed rest and, in some cases, sedation to prevent movement of the eye, which can cause re-bleeding. If the bleeding does not resolve, it can stain the corneal endothelium. It can also cause secondary glaucoma by blocking the aqueous drainage. Surgical removal of the clotted blood may be necessary.

Corneal Ulcer

This is a very serious condition caused by erosion and infection of the cornea. It can produce permanent scarring and blindness. The infecting agent can be bacterial or fungal or both. This is an emergency and early identification of the organism(s) will reduce or prevent serious scarring.

The common bacterial agents include: Staphylococcus, Streptococcus pneumonia, Haemophilus and Moraxella. Pseudomonas and Klebsiella are less common but are much more destructive.

Diagnosis

Pus is usually associated with a corneal ulcer. The ulcer can occur anywhere on the cornea and appears as a yellowish or whitish depression or defect. The patient usually complains of pain, loss of vision and tearing. The entire eye looks very inflamed with injection of the blood vessels. In severe cases, hypopyon (abnormal cells) may be present in the anterior chamber.

A patient with a corneal ulcer should be under the care of an ophthalmologist. If that is not possible, consultation should be done remotely under the guidance of the ophthalmologist, and the patient should be admitted to the hospital for intense topical antibiotic and/or antifungal treatment.

The eye should not be patched, as patching an infected eye would only make it warmer, darker and more moist, all of which would make the infection worse.

Herpes Simplex Keratitis

This is a serious condition. The virus initially infects the corneal and conjunctival epithelium, and can invade deep into the corneal stroma. Secondary bacterial infection may occur and can lead to corneal perforation and permanent blindness. Dense corneal scarring can occur in some herpes simplex infections.

The diagnosis can be made by the telltale dendritic (branching) pattern of corneal epithelial defect when examined with the aid of fluorescein dye. Other staining patterns may also occur.
Topical corticosteroids should never be used to treat this condition. It can lead to deeper invasion by the virus, worsening the infection.

The treatment is ganciclovir 0.15% ophthalmic gel, trifluridine 1% (Viroptic) or vidarabine 3% ointment. Oral anti-viral agents (acyclovir 400 mg p.o. five times per day for 7 to 10 days) may be prescribed to avoid the toxicity of topical anti-viral drops or when drops cannot be given, such as when treating children.
When no anti-viral agent is available, treatment with an antibiotic drop or ointment should be given to prevent secondary bacterial infection.

Pterygium

Pterygium is a conjunctival growth extending onto the cornea, usually on the nasal side. It is more frequent in sunny, hot, dry and dusty places. If the growth begins to encroach on the visual axis, it should be surgically removed. The recurrence rate used to be high, but now, with the help of antimetabolite drugs, recurrence is less frequent.

SCLERA

Scleritis

This is an inflammation of the sclera and may be a sign of system disease such as rheumatoid arthritis. The patient usually complains of an aching pain in the eye, and the eyeball is usually tender to the touch. The lesion is pinkish and seems to lie deep in the conjunctiva. Vision is usually not affected.

Topical corticosteroid is the treatment. The patient should be followed closely to watch for complications of the corticosteroid, and it should be stopped as quickly as possible. Non-steroidal anti-inflammatory drugs may be substituted to prevent exacerbation of the condition. Chronic scleritis can lead to scleral thinning.

CHAPTER 6: CATARACT

Cataract is defined as any opacity in the natural crystalline lens.

Anatomy of the Crystalline Lens

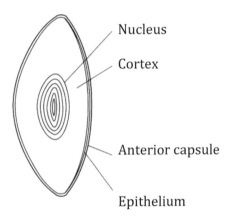

- The crystalline lens is enclosed by a clear elastic membrane.
- The anterior capsule sits immediately behind the iris.
- The epithelium is a layer of cells beneath the anterior capsule.
- The cortex is a clear protein substance inside the capsule.
- The nucleus is the center of the lens.
- The posterior capsule faces the vitreous.

When we are young, the nucleus is soft. As we get older, it becomes progressively harder.

It is generally believed that excessive exposure to ultraviolet light can cause cataract, as demonstrated by the high incidence of the condition in countries close to the equator and at high altitudes. Poor nutrition and smoking may be contributing factors in the development of cataract, and certain drugs such as corticosteroids, either oral or topical, can also cause the disease. Some other well-known causes include trauma, diabetes mellitus, and inflammation.

In addition, cataract can be congenital secondary to metabolic diseases such as galactosemia. Fetal infection with the rubella virus before the ninth week of gestation can also cause the disorder.

A patient with a cataract will complain of blurry vision. The cataract can be seen easily with a slit lamp; or a pocket flashlight or direct ophthalmoscope can be used to detect the opacity as well. If the lens appears cloudy, a cataract is present. In early stages, before surgery is indicated, primary care physicians should recommend that their patients follow a healthy diet, exercise, avoid smoking, and protect their eyes from UV light. Once a cataract is suspected, the patient should be referred to an optometrist or ophthalmologist for further evaluation.

Surgical Treatment of Cataract

When I did my ophthalmology residency in the late 1970s, we almost entirely performed intracapsular cataract extraction (ICCE) for the treatment of cataract. This is the removal of the entire lens, usually with a cryoprobe. The probe is connected to a cryo (freezing) machine, which makes it extremely cold, and when the probe touches the lens, the lens becomes an ice ball and is then removed from the eye.

The problem with this method was that it had many potential complications, some of which were severe. The anterior chamber IOL (intraocular lens) implanted after the lens removal also caused many complications. Patients were usually fitted with thick spectacles following surgery, which caused them to see objects about 30% larger. They had to be careful getting around, as they had to learn to judge their new spatial relationship.

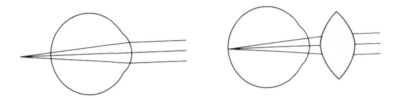

Aphakic vision without correction is like being blind (left). Correction with thick glasses makes the image about 30% larger (right).

When I began my practice in the early 1980s, the **extracapsular (ECCE) method** was gaining popularity. This had many advantages over the ICCE because it required a smaller incision. Only the opaque portions of the lens were removed. The integrity of the posterior capsule and anterior vitreous face were not disturbed. This significantly reduced the incidence of complications, which included retinal detachment and cystoid macular edema (CME).

With the ECCE method, intraocular lenses had become much safer because they could now sit on the posterior capsule away from the vascular structures in the anterior chamber.

ECCE Method

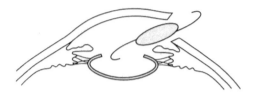

- The anterior capsule is opened and removed.
- The hard nucleus is removed.
- The loose cortex is then removed by aspiration/irrigation.
- The posterior capsule remains intact.
- The IOL is placed inside the capsular bag, resting on the posterior capsule.

The **phacoemulsification method** (using ultra sonic energy to remove the cataract before placing the IOL) is now generally used in developed countries. In developing countries, most cataract surgeries are done with the ECCE method, which has proven to be just as safe and effective as the phacoemulsification method. The phacoemulsification method is more expensive, as it is done with an expensive machine, and extra costs are incurred in each case with disposable supplies such as tubing and fluid.

Cataract surgery with **femtosecond laser** is a new method of removing the cataract using ultra-fast energy pulses to break apart the cataract at the molecular level. This involves a machine even more expensive than the phacoemulsification machine. The majority of cataract surgeries in the US are done using the phacoemulsification method.

When should the cataract be removed?

It depends on the visual needs of the patient. When the vision is blurry enough to interfere with activities of daily living such as reading print and seeing signs while driving, surgery should be considered. In the US, the DMV requires 20/40 vision in at least one eye for a driver's license, although sometimes exceptions may be made following a driving test. Some professions, such as airline pilots, require better vision.

Cataract surgery is one of the safest surgical procedures, and up to 95% of patients will find an improvement in their vision. However, it is a surgery and it carries some risks. Infection is very rare, about 1 to 2 in a thousand, but when it occurs, it can be very serious.

Congenital cataracts should be treated as soon as possible to prevent amblyopia (lazy eye). When a baby is born, the eyes have to learn to work with the brain in order to see. If the vision is blocked by a cataract, the eye is unable to send clear images to the brain and it may never learn to see clearly. When that child becomes an adult, even after the cataract is removed, the vision would still be very blurry.

CHAPTER 7: RETINA AND VITREOUS

This is an exciting time to be a retina specialist because we have so many more options for treatment. When I finished my fellowship in the early 1980s and began my practice, laser had only been used to treat diabetic retinopathy for a few years. There was essentially no treatment for macular degeneration. In the early 2000s, a new class of drug called anti-VEGF was available for treatment in macular degeneration, and this totally revolutionized the management of this disabling disease.

Primary care doctors need to know the most common retinal conditions so that they can make appropriate and timely referrals. Any abnormality observed in the retina should be referred to an ophthalmologist. Practice with the ophthalmoscope will make recognizing the difference between normal and abnormal easier with time.

DIABETIC RETINOPATHY

Diabetes mellitus can be such a devastating disease because it can affect almost every organ in the body, especially those with small blood vessels such as the eye, the kidneys and the peripheral nerves.

Diabetic retinopathy is one of the top causes of blindness all over the world. With developing countries becoming more prosperous and the people taking in more calories, there has been a drastic increase in diabetes mellitus among these populations. When I spent two weeks in Western Samoa in 2014 treating patients, I was distressed to see so many people coming into the clinic with advanced diabetic retinopathy. Some of the eyes were beyond laser treatment and went blind. The incidence of diabetes in Western Samoa is between 20% and 25%. In China, which we don't usually associate with a high rate of diabetes, I was surprised to learn that the incidence of the disease has gone up to 10% in recent years.

The duration of diabetes is the major risk factor in the appearance of diabetic retinopathy. After 25 years as a diabetic, a patient has a 26% chance of developing the severe form of retinopathy, the proliferative type that can cause blindness without treatment.

Pathogenesis:
After prolonged periods of exposure to high levels of glucose, the capillaries are damaged from the loss of intramural pericytes. The blood-retinal barrier is compromised, leading to capillary closure. If the capillary closure is extensive, it can lead to the production of a chemical substance called **VEGF** (Vascular Endothelial Growth Factor). As capillary closure causes hypoxia, the body tries to grow new vessels to repair the damage. Unfortunately, this can cause serious complications in the eye. Instead of helping the hypoxia, the production of new vessels can bleed inside the eye or go on to fibrosis, pulling on the retina and leading to retinal detachment.

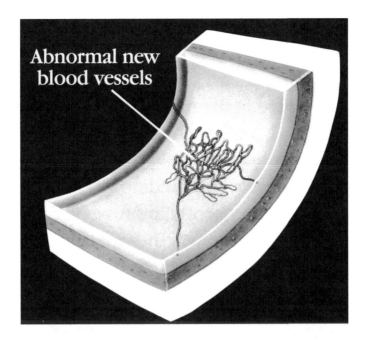

Abnormal new vessels on the retinal surface, caused by hypoxia in the tissue, which produces VEGF and stimulates the growth of neovascularization. These abnormal vessels can cause bleeding in the eye. If not treated with laser, they can go on to fibrosis and cause traction retinal detachment.

Blindness is the end result of untreated neovascularization.

Management:
Good control of the patient's glucose levels will reduce the severity of the retinopathy.

Hypertension is associated with 20% of diabetics, and the elevated blood pressure can further complicate a retinopathy.

Treatment:

Laser treatment has proven to be a very effective treatment for diabetic retinopathy. By destroying the neovascularization, the complication of bleeding into the eye is eliminated, and the vessels are also prevented from going on to the fibrotic stage. By destroying part of the retina that is less important for our vision, we save the central retina, i.e., the area around the macula that is essential. Once the sick retinal vessels are destroyed, they no longer require oxygen. This helps the hypoxic situation and prevents further release of VEGF and the production of neovascularization.

TYPES OF DIABETES

Type I (juvenile onset)

This is believed to be an autoimmune disease, usually triggered by an illness that leads to the destruction of the insulin-producing cells in the pancreas. This group has a high risk for developing severe proliferative retinopathy.

Type II (adult onset)

The majority of patients with diabetes belong to this group. It is caused by insulin-resistant receptor cells. The insulin level is usually normal and can even be elevated.

TYPES OF DIABETIC RETINOPATHY

1. Background retinopathy (non-proliferative): This is an early stage of retina damage caused by constricting capillaries in diabetics. The patient's vision will not be affected at this stage. Findings include intra-retinal hemorrhages, dilated veins, hard exudates, microaneurysms, retinal edema, CWS (Cotton Wool Spots) and dot-blot hemorrhages.

2. Pre-proliferative retinopathy: This is the most severe stage of background retinopathy in which symptoms have increased in severity, but new vessels are not yet forming. It can include venous beading, a significant indicator that these patients will likely go on to the proliferative stage.

3. Proliferative diabetic retinopathy: This occurs in 5% of patients with diabetic retinopathy. New blood vessels (neovascularization) grow on the surface of the retina and the optic nerve, and sometimes into the vitreous. This can lead to vitreous hemorrhage and/or traction retinal detachment.

4. Diabetic maculopathy: This finding may be seen in any phase of retinopathy except the very early phase of background retinopathy. Macular edema builds up due to increased vascular permeability, whereby the blood vessels leak fluid onto the macula.

LASER TREATMENT

This is usually done in the office and takes from 15 to 30 minutes, depending on the type and extent of the treatment. Only topical anesthetics are required in most cases.

In proliferative diabetic retinopathy, pan-retinal photocoagulation (PRP) is needed. This usually requires more than one session. In one session, up to 500 laser spots may be applied to the peripheral retina.

In macular edema secondary to any phase of the retinopathy, small focal laser spots are applied to discrete areas of leakage.

Low power laser spots may be applied in a grid pattern to areas of diffuse leakage.

Laser treatment for diabetic retinopathy is one of the safest and most effective treatments in medicine. It does not improve the vision, and the best it can do is preserve the existing vision. One of the side effects of extensive laser treatment is decreased night vision.

Without laser treatment, a person with severe proliferative diabetic retinopathy will eventually go blind. In the 21st century, with laser treatment readily available in most countries, there is no reason why a person with diabetes should go blind.

Every diabetic patient should be educated about the disease's complications, especially those relating to the eye. Depending on the duration and severity of the diabetes, or if diabetic retinopathy is already present, the patient should have eye examinations at regular intervals, such as once a year.

The patient should see an ophthalmologist if there is any sudden change in vision, such as distortion in the central vision or sudden onset of floaters.

Pan-retinal laser photocoagulation (PRP) for treatment of proliferative diabetic retinopathy (PDR)

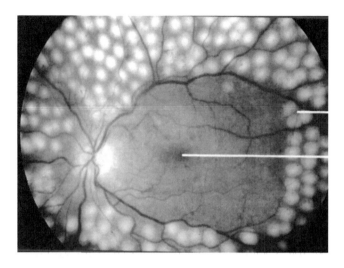

Each spot is a laser burn. This area of the retina has been destroyed and no longer requires oxygen, thus alleviating the hypoxic condition. No new blood vessels will grow after such a treatment.

The area around the macula is spared. With this area intact, the reading vision will remain the same. Night vision may be decreased after an extensive treatment.

MACULAR DEGENERATION

AMD or age-related macular degeneration is grouped into dry and wet forms. AMD is the main cause of loss of vision in patients over 50 years old in the US and Western Europe. It is a disease mainly found in light-complexioned persons and sometimes can be inherited. But the pattern of inheritance is rarely proven.

Dry AMD

Drusen (yellow deposits deep in the retina) and atrophy of the RPE (retinal pigment epithelium) are associated with this form of AMD. It can cause loss of vision if the atrophy involves the center of the macula.

The Age-Related Eye Disease Study (AREDS) showed that patients with dry AMD could reduce the risk of visual loss by taking high doses of vitamins and zinc. Commercially prepared combinations of vitamins and minerals for this purpose are available.

Wet AMD

In this condition, the retina and RPE are detached from the underlying structures by serous fluid. The space under the RPE is invaded by abnormal blood vessels from the choroid forming the choroidal neovascular membrane (CNV), which can bleed. These hemorrhages eventually form fibrovascular diskiform scars, which are often in the macular area, leading to severe loss of vision.

A **fluorescein angiogram** showing a CNV (choroidal neovascular membrane) in the macula.

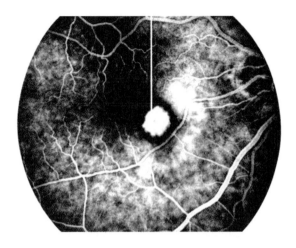

A fluorescein angiography is done by injecting the fluorescent dye into the bloodstream, highlighting the blood vessels in the back of the eye so they can be photographed.

Patients with either form of AMD should be instructed to test their own eyes with the Amsler grid. If any distortion of the lines is noted, the patient should see a retina specialist as soon as possible.

Treatment of Wet AMD

Until the early 2000s, there was no effective treatment for wet AMD, i.e., the CNV that causes the damage. For the occasional CNVs that are not inside the macula, we would try to destroy them with laser treatment. But they often returned and eventually extended into the macula. Now we have a new class of drug called anti-VEGF that can block the chemical that causes the CNV to form in the first place, preventing further loss of vision.

Anti-VEGF Therapy

VEGF stimulates the formation of CNV, and by blocking the effect of this protein, it is prevented from further stimulating the growth of CNV.

There are several anti-VEGF drugs on the market. Lucentis (ranibizumab) is the first to be approved by the FDA for the treatment of wet macular degeneration.

The drug is injected directly into the vitreous, which then diffuses throughout the retina and choroid. By binding strongly to the VEGF proteins, it prevents further growth of unwanted blood vessels. It has been touted as the miracle drug for macular degeneration because, for so long, there was essentially no treatment. For the majority of patients, the drug stops the disease from progressing. In some patients, there is actually a small gain of vision. This treatment is time consuming, as the injection has to be done almost monthly. It is also expensive, each dose costing about $2,000.

Avastin (bevacizumab) was developed for the treatment of metastatic colon cancer. It has a similar but larger molecular structure than Lucentis. The two drugs are manufactured by the same company. Avastin has been widely used for the treatment of wet AMD by many ophthalmologists in the US, even though the FDA has not approved it to date. It has been determined to be just as effective and safe as Lucentis. The cost of each dose of this drug is about $50, i.e., 2.5% of the price of Lucentis.

So why do ophthalmologists still use Lucentis? This is a hotly debated, complicated issue. Those of you who are interested may get on the Internet for further reading.

FLASHES AND FLOATERS

When we are young, the vitreous is a clear jell-like substance with millions of fine fibers. As we get older, it shrinks, and part of it becomes liquefied, causing a **posterior vitreous detachment**. The tugging of the vitreous where it is attached to the retina causes the brain to interpret this as flashes of light. This process also causes the formation of strands and strings appearing as spots, small circles or fine threads floating inside the eye. Most of the time, there is no real threat to the vision and the patient will learn to live with these floaters. If they are severe enough, some retinal specialists might recommend their removal with vitrectomy (surgical removal of the vitreous). This form of treatment is controversial and is not generally accepted as standard procedure.

RETINAL TEAR

In some areas, the vitreous may be very strongly attached to the retina. If these areas happen to contain weak or thin retina, a piece of it can be torn off. If there is a blood vessel across the tear, bleeding may occur. This is called a **vitreous hemorrhage**. If there is a great deal of hemorrhage, it may reduce the vision.

If a retinal tear occurs, it can be a serious problem, as it can go on to a retinal detachment. A retinal tear can be treated with laser photocoagulation or cryo therapy. The area treated will form a scar around the tear, which will prevent the retina from detaching.

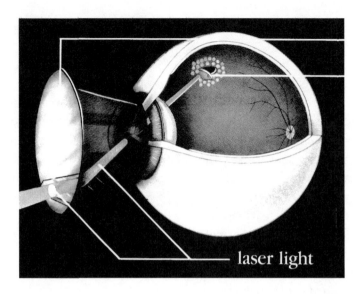

laser light

This is a so-called "horseshoe" tear because it is shaped like a horseshoe.

The patient sits in front of the slit lamp. A special contact lens is placed on the cornea.

The laser is applied around the edges of the tear in two or three rows.

A firm adhesion forms around the tear, preventing a detached retina.

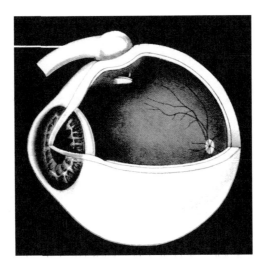

The same retinal tear can also be treated by cryo therapy.

Under direct visualization, the cryo probe is placed under the area of the retinal tear.

An ice ball forms, freezing the area around the tear, creating an adhesion and preventing the tear from becoming a detached retina.

RETINAL DETACHMENT

When fluid collects in the potential space between the sensory retina and RPE, it becomes a detached retina. There are several types of retinal detachment. Here we will only discuss the rhegmatogenous type, which is invariably caused by a retinal hole or tear (break) in the retina.

This type of retinal detachment occurs more frequently in people with myopia or after trauma, such as in the case of boxers.

The symptom would be loss of side vision, which many patients describe as a curtain. If the macula is also detached, then the central vision would be lost as well.

If the detached retina has a large amount of fluid underneath it, it would be recognizable by its marked elevation. The detached retina appears opaque and may undulate. It is very difficult to examine a detached retina with a handheld ophthalmoscope. Ophthalmologists use the indirect ophthalmoscope, which provides stereopsis and an entire 360-degree view of the retina including the extreme periphery, which is the usual location of a retinal hole or tear. The first thing in the repair of a detached retina is to find the hole(s) or tear(s), which have to be sealed in order to have a successful outcome.

Repair of Retinal Detachment

Until about two decades ago, the usual treatment for retinal detachment was the scleral buckling procedure. As the technology for vitrectomy improves, become less invasive and involves fewer complications, most detached retina surgeries done in the US now use the vitrectomy method.

The **scleral buckling procedure** is still very useful, especially in developing countries where the very expensive vitrectomy machine is not available. I have done scleral buckling procedures in several developing countries with supplies that I brought with me. The only additional supply I needed was a tank of gas (carbon dioxide or nitrous oxide are available in most developing countries) for the portable cryo machine. A portable laser (which I often bring along as well) can also be used to treat the retinal tear.

A piece of silicone sponge is sutured onto the sclera over the area of the retinal tear. This creates an indentation, pushing the choroid against the retina at the location of the tear. The tear is then treated with cryo therapy to cause an inflammation that encourages an adhesion to form between the retina and choroid.

Depending on the size and location of the retinal tear, the silicone sponge can be trimmed to fit the size requirements of the area to be treated.

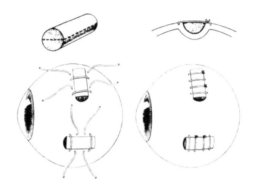

All retinal breaks are localized and treated with cryo therapy. A silicone sponge is then sutured to the sclera, making an indentation that pushes the choroid against the retina. The fluid underneath the retina is resorbed by the RPE. The area treated with the cryo therapy forms a chorioretinal adhesion.

Pneumatic retinopexy is used in select cases where the retinal detachment is limited and the tear is in a superior location. In these cases, a gas bubble is injected into the vitreous cavity. The patient is then positioned so that the gas pushes the retina around the break, creating a tamponade and sealing the tear. The area around the tear is then treated with cyro therapy or laser. After 1 to 2 weeks, the special gas, which is usually SF6 (sulfur hexafluoride), is resorbed and disappears from the eye. By then, a chorioretinal adhesion would have formed to keep the retina attached.

In **vitrectomy**, the vitreous pulling on the retinal break is removed. A gas bubble is usually injected to push the retina around the break against the choroid. In more complicated detached retinas, more extensive surgery such as removal of scar tissue on the retina may be needed.

A vitrectomy is performed under microscopic control by inserting tiny instruments (25 or 27 gauge) through the pars plana of the eye. This is an area of the sclera behind the limbus and is usually avascular. Visualization inside the eye is made possible with fiber-optic illumination. Instruments that can perform vitreous cutting and aspiration and tiny scissors are used. A tiny fiber-optic probe attached to a laser machine can be inserted into the eye for laser photocoagulation during the surgery under direct visualization.

Vitrectomy is used for other indications such as non-resolving vitreous hemorrhage and penetrating injuries to the eyeball.

OCCLUSIONS

Central Retinal Artery Occlusion (CRAO)—also included in the neuro-ophthalmology chapter.

CRAO is manifested as a sudden loss of vision. Prolonged (over 45 minutes) interruption of retinal arterial blood flow causes permanent damage to the ganglion and other cells, resulting in permanent loss of vision. The typical feature is a so-called "cherry-red spot."

Branch Retinal Artery Occlusion (BRAO)

When only a branch of the central retinal artery is involved, the area of the retina supplied by this branch becomes ischemic with a corresponding loss of vision in the visual field.

Central Retinal Vein Occlusion (CRVO)

The fundus picture of CRVO is dramatic, with acute hemorrhages and disc swelling, the so-called "blood and thunder" picture. Visual loss is usually not acute and the condition is not an emergency; there is generally no accepted acute management. The hemorrhages and disc swelling may improve with time, along with improvement of the vision.

This condition is most often found in older people with hypertension and arteriosclerotic vascular disease. Carotid artery occlusion may produce similar but less severe findings.

Neovascular glaucoma can be a late complication of CRVO. Laser photocoagulation can prevent this complication.

Branch Retinal Vein Occlusion (BRVO)

Obstruction of outflow can cause retinal vein occlusion, which in turn causes edema, abnormal leakage and hemorrhage to the area of the retina involved.

Prolonged obstruction can cause ischemia, which in turn can lead to the growth of neovascularization. Again, neovascularization, if allowed to proliferate untreated (with laser photocoagulation), can lead to vitreous hemorrhage and traction retinal detachment.

CHAPTER 8: UVEITIS

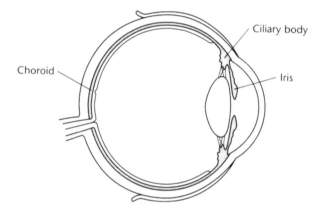

The uveal tract includes the iris, ciliary body and choroid. The primary function of the uveal tract is to supply nourishment to the ocular structures.

Uveitis is a general term for inflammation of the uveal tract, i.e., iritis, cyclitis (inflammation of the ciliary body), irido-cyclitis and choroiditis.

Uveitis is a difficult area even for ophthalmologists, because it is not easy to pinpoint the cause, and often extensive studies are required. Frequently, the adjacent structures such as retina, sclera and cornea are also involved secondary to the inflammatory process.

Uveitis is divided into 3 types: anterior, intermediate and posterior.

In this book, we will concentrate mainly on the anterior variety, as it is the most common and can be treated at most medical clinics.

Symptoms of Uveitis:
- Redness
- Pain
- Photophobia
- Tearing
- Visual disturbance
- Floaters

Anterior uveitis can be acute or chronic. Blunt trauma to the eyeball can cause anterior uveitis with acute onset of pain, hyperemia, photophobia and blurry vision. The pupil is miotic. Flare (a foggy appearance) and cells (WBCs) are found in the anterior chamber, which can only be seen with the slit lamp under high magnification.

Some Causes of Anterior Uveitis:
- Idiopathic
- Traumatic
- Juvenile rheumatoid arthritis
- Sarcoidosis
- Syphilis
- AIDS
- Tuberculosis

Treatment is corticosteroid drops (for the inflammation) and dilation of the pupil with a cycloplegic drop to relax the ciliary muscle. Corticosteroids should be used with great caution because of their serious side effects. If the condition is not resolved in less than a week, the patient should be sent to an ophthalmologist.

Some diseases involve more than one segment.

Some Causes of **Intermediate Uveitis**:
- Idiopathic
- Lyme disease
- Sarcoidosis
- Multiple sclerosis
- Juvenile rheumatoid arthritis

Some Causes of **Posterior Uveitis**:
- Idiopathic
- Toxoplasmosis
- Sarcoidosis
- AIDS
- Candidiasis

Some Causes of **Panuveitis** (involving the entire uveal tract):
- Idiopathic
- Sarcoidosis
- Vogt-Koyanagi-Harada
- Behcet syndrome

Panuveitis tends to be a chronic disease with a fair to poor prognosis.

Except for mild anterior uveitis, patients should be referred to an ophthalmologist. This can be a blinding disease.

The lists of causes are far from complete, as I have chosen to include only diseases that primary care practitioners are generally familiar with. Treatment of severe uveitis is beyond the scope of this book.

CHAPTER 9: GLAUCOMA

Glaucoma is a group of diseases that damages the optic nerve. At its simplest and most useful for the purposes of this book, glaucoma is a condition in which the optic nerve has been damaged by elevated intraocular pressure.

The normal range of IOP (intraocular pressure) is between 10-21 mm Hg. In some eyes, damage can occur within this range. When that happens, it is called "low tension" or "normotensive" glaucoma. An IOP of over 21 mm Hg does not always mean that the nerve will be damaged.

The anterior chamber of the eye contains aqueous fluid, which is constantly produced by the ciliary body. In a healthy eye (below), the fluid drains out of the eyeball through the trabecular meshwork located at the periphery of the anterior chamber just anterior to the iris.

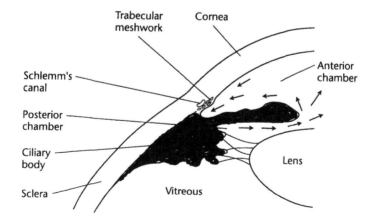

The "angle" discussed in glaucoma diagnoses consists of the base of the iris, the trabecular meshwork and the supporting scleral and corneal tissue. If the production of the fluid exceeds the outflow, the IOP rises.

PRIMARY OPEN-ANGLE GLAUCOMA

This is the most common type of glaucoma, usually found in older people. As people age, the trabecular meshwork becomes less efficient and IOP builds up. As its name implies, the angle between the base of the iris, trabecular meshwork and the supporting scleral and corneal tissue is open. It is usually bilateral and may be inherited. Good central vision is usually preserved until late in the disease, which makes this type of glaucoma very dangerous, as it is initially asymptomatic unless visual field testing is done.

Patients with advanced glaucoma may have difficulty getting around because of the constricted visual field.

Examination of the optic nerve may reveal enlarged cupping and its color can appear less pink than normal.

THE OPTIC NERVE

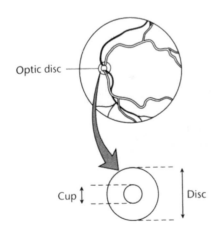

Optic disc

Cup   Disc

The healthy optic nerve is pinkish in color. The center of the optic nerve (physiologic optic cup) or the cup/disc ratio is usually 30% or less of the diameter of the optic disc.

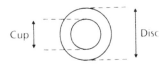

The cup/disc ratio here is 0.6. The pinkish nerve tissue, especially on the temporal side of the optic disc, may be damaged and thin.
Glaucoma is suspected.

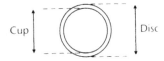

The cup/disc ratio is 0.9 here. The optic cup becomes whitish and deeper. Tiny hemorrhages may appear on the optic disc.

For a patient with a cup/disc ratio of 0.9, the visual field is usually severely constricted.

There are various visual field machines, some of which are very sensitive, that can detect early loss of peripheral vision.

VISUAL FIELDS

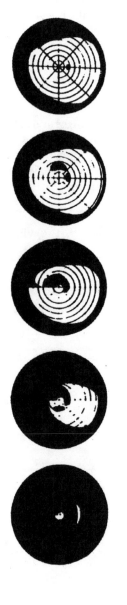

This is a normal visual field.
Cup/disc ratio is 0.3.

Field shows enlarged blind spot and superior nasal scotoma. In glaucoma, the cup usually enlarges more vertically.
Cup/disc ratio is 0.5 horizontally and 0.6 vertically.

Field shows constriction of superior nasal field. There is thinning of the rim of the cup.
Cup/disc ratio is 0.8.

Field shows further superior constriction and new inferior defect. Cup/disc ratio is 0.9 with advanced generalized thinning of the rim.

Field shows small central and temporal island of vision remaining. The optic nerve is pale with a deep cup and total atrophy of the rim.

CROSS-CONFRONTATION VISUAL FIELD TESTING

1. Sit facing the patient, about 3 feet away.
2. Cover the patient's left eye with a patch.
3. Have the patient's right eye visually fix on your nose.
4. Test the right eye by holding your left hand outside of the patient's visual field. Slowly move your hand (with an arbitrary number of fingers) from the patient's temporal side. Ask the patient to tell you when he/she can first count the number of fingers. Repeat this step for the superior temporal and inferior temporal quadrants. Switch hands and check the superior nasal and inferior nasal quadrants. Map your findings onto a rough visual field chart.
5. Cover the right eye and test the left.

This visual field test can also be used for patients with neurological problems such as pituitary gland tumor.

MEDICAL TREATMENT

The goal of glaucoma treatment is to prevent further damage to the optic nerve and retina. The desired IOP may vary from patient to patient. Medical treatment is usually life long and requires the diligence and cooperation of the patient.

Medications

Cholinergic-stimulating drugs:
Miotics help to drain the aqueous through the trabecular meshwork more rapidly. Pilocarpine 1% to 6%, one drop topically every 6 hours, may be prescribed. Pilocarpine gel is also available.

Because of its side effects and the availability of better drugs, it is no longer a common drug for the treatment of primary open-angle glaucoma. Its side effects include blurry vision, frontal headaches, and sometimes nausea.

Beta blockers (beta-adrenergic blocking agents):
These reduce the IOP by reducing aqueous production by the ciliary body. Timoptic (timolol maleate) was the first beta blocker to be approved for treatment of glaucoma. It is usually used twice a day. One daily dose is effective for 70% of patients. Beta-blockers are usually excellent for lowering IOP.

Patients with asthma, chronic lung disease and congestive heart failure should not use this group of medication.

Other beta-blockers: Betagan, Betoptic-S, Optipranolol, Ocupress.

Prostaglandin inhibitors:
Xalatan (Latanoprost), a prostaglandin inhibitor, lowers the IOP by increasing the aqueous fluid outflow by a pathway other than the meshwork. It is very expensive and requires refrigeration.
Other prostaglandin inhibitors: Lumigan, Travatan, Rescula.

Alpha-adrenergic agonists:
These drugs lower the IOP by decreasing the aqueous production. They are: Iopidine (apraclonidine) and Alphagan (brimonidine).

Adrenergic stimulating drugs:
Epinephrine hydrochloride and Propine (dipivefrin).

Carbonic anhydrase inhibitors:
Diamox (Acetazolamide) lowers the IOP by decreasing aqueous production by the ciliary body. It is widely available in oral form, 250 mg every 6 hours or 500 mg sequel every 12 hours. It is

rarely used for the treatment of chronic glaucoma in oral form because of the side effects, which include kidney stones, body chemistry disturbance (loss of potassium), gastrointestinal upsets, loss of appetite and weight loss.

Other carbonic anhydrase inhibitors: Neptazane (methazolamide) and Daranide (dichlorphenamide).

Topical carbonic anhydrase inhibitors: Trusopt (dorzolamide) and Azopt (brinzolamide).

Combination drops:
Cosopt = (timolol + dorzolamide)
Combigan = (timolol + brimonidine)

Hyperosmotics:
Glycerin (glycerol) may be given orally to dehydrate the vitreous and lower the IOP. Mannitol and urea are intravenous hyperosmotics. These agents are usually used in a hospital setting.

SURGICAL MANAGEMENT

When medical or laser treatments fail, or when they become impractical, surgery should be considered.

In the UK, surgery is often undertaken early in glaucoma treatment instead of committing the patient to a life of drugs that can be inconvenient and expensive. In the US, possibly because of fear of lawsuits, surgery is only offered as a very last resort.

Laser Trabeculoplasty

Using a high-intensity beam of light (laser), several evenly spaced tiny burns are made in the trabecular meshwork, allowing the aqueous to drain better, lowering the pressure.

Only topical anesthesia is needed for this usually painless procedure, which takes about 15 minutes. The drop in IOP is not typically very great after such a procedure, and the patient may still need to use medicated drops.

Trabeculectomy

This is the most common external filtration surgery. A tiny section of the sclera and trabecular meshwork at the limbus is removed. The opening is then covered with a loosely sutured scleral flap, and the area is recovered with the conjunctiva. The aqueous flows through the fistula under the conjunctiva, creating a bleb. If the surgery works well, the IOP becomes normal because of the constant flow of aqueous leaving the eyeball.

This procedure is not done more frequently in the US because of potential complications such as wound leakage and prolonged low IOP. The most dreaded complication is infection (endophthalmitis).

Trabeculectomy

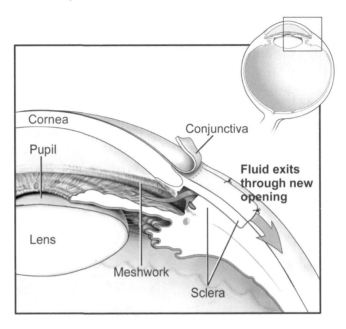

- A tiny block of sclera and trabecular meshwork is removed.
- The opening is covered with a loosely sutured scleral flap.
- Aqueous flows through a fistula.
- A bleb (small rounded mound) is created under the conjunctiva.
- A constant amount of aqueous leaves the eye, normalizing the IOP.

PRIMARY ANGLE-CLOSURE GLAUCOMA

When the iris suddenly blocks the trabecular meshwork, interrupting the outflow of aqueous, it causes a marked increase in the IOP, which can cause pain and decrease vision. It is usually bilateral, but acute attacks of angle-closure do not typically occur at the same time. This condition is most common among Asians, because of their typically smaller eyes (i.e., narrower angle), and uncommon in people of African descent, because they often have larger eyes (i.e., wider angle).

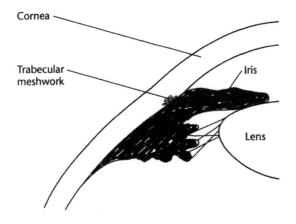

The iris is up against the angle, blocking the trabecular meshwork, stopping the aqueous fluid from leaving the eye. The sudden rise of IOP can cause pain, loss of vision and colored rings or halos around lights. The pain can be very severe. The loss of vision is secondary to the corneal edema from the high IOP.

The IOP may be as high as 50 to 60 mm Hg. Palpation of the eyeball over the upper eyelid will feel firm.

In an acute attack, medical therapy should be initiated as soon as possible because the elevated IOP can cause permanent damage to the optic nerve.

Medical Treatment of Acute Angle Closure

1. Pilocarpine 4% drop every half hour until the pupil constricts.
2. Beta-blocker such as Timolol Maleate 0.5%, one drop every 10 minutes until the IOP is lowered to an acceptable level.
3. Diamox 500 mg orally.
4. Glycerin 50% solution given orally, 1.5 g per kg of body weight.

Laser Iridotomy or Surgical Iridectomy

Once the IOP and inflammation have been brought under control, and the cornea is clear, a laser iridotomy should be done as soon as possible. Laser iridotomy (using the laser to burn a hole in the iris) can be done in the office and is much safer than surgical iridectomy. Either an argon laser or Nd:YAG laser can be used to make this opening.

Surgical iridectomy (surgical removal of a tiny piece of peripheral iris near the angle) may be needed if the iridotomy keeps closing off or when the laser is not available. It involves cutting into the eye and carries the risks and complication of a delicate surgery.

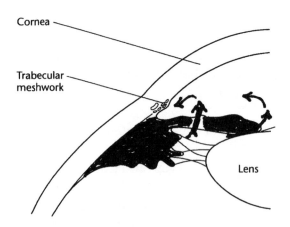

Cornea

Trabecular meshwork

Lens

Creating an opening in the peripheral iris allows the aqueous fluid to flow from the posterior chamber to the anterior chamber. This will keep the iris from bulging forward to block off the trabecular meshwork.

The unaffected eye will generally benefit from a prophylactic laser iridotomy or surgical iridectomy; otherwise, it will be a matter of time before it suffers an angle-closure attack as well.

SECONDARY GLAUCOMA

Systemic diseases such as diabetes can cause the dreaded neovascular glaucoma, which can be very painful and can lead to blindness.

Advanced cataract or a dislocated lens can cause the IOP to go up.

Uveitis (inflammation inside the eye) can cause an acute rise in IOP.

Injury to the eye can cause the IOP to go up in different ways.

GLAUCOMA IN DEVELOPING COUNTRIES

If a patient in a developing country has chronic glaucoma, it would be difficult for him or her to shoulder the cost of a lifetime of medication and the follow-up needed for such a condition. The patient may live far away from any medical facility, and may not understand the natural history of the disease.

Glaucoma is a difficult disease to manage when trying to make a living is a problem. Early surgery would be recommended. Otherwise, these patients will almost certainly go blind, as it is unlikely that they will consistently follow the daily routine of applying the necessary eye drop(s).

CHAPTER 10: NEURO-OPHTHALMOLOGY

The process of human vision is incredibly complex. There are two main components: the eye, which is responsible for collecting information, and the brain, which is responsible for interpreting it. The eye is like a camera, and all the parts have to be in good condition for a clear image to form on the retina. If any part of the eye, such as the cornea, the lens, the vitreous or the retina, is not perfect, then a clear image cannot be obtained.

The image captured by the retina is converted to electrochemical signals, which are then sent along the axons of the ganglion cells in the retina. The ganglion cells all meet to form the optic nerve, which is also known as the optic disc.

Please refer to the Visual-Sensory System and Visual Pathway diagrams on pages 93-94.

Fibers from the macula enter the temporal side of the optic disc. After perforating the sclera, the optic nerve fibers pass directly to the optic chiasm.

Fibers from the nasal halves of each retina cross to the other side. Optic fibers from the temporal halves of each retina move toward the chiasm, leaving it without crossing. The optic fibers behind the chiasm form the optic tract, which goes to the geniculate body (the right and left) of the thalamus.

The fibers in front of the chiasm are called the optic nerves and those behind are the optic tracts.

The visual sensory information is sent to the occipital lobe (the visual cortex) to be interpreted. From the visual cortex, the visual sensory information is simultaneously sent to the "what" and "where" pathways, which are located primarily in the temporal lobe and parietal lobe, respectively.

The "what" pathway is a pattern recognition center, which we develop from the time we are babies, learning forms, shapes and faces in our surroundings. Initially, babies make little sense of the world around them, but gradually they become familiar with their environments.

The book The Man Who Mistook His Wife for a Hat *is about a man who has trouble recognizing his students until they speak to him. This is an example of brain damage in the "what" pathway, whereby he is no longer able to recognize objects that used to be familiar to him.*

The "where" pathway, located in the parietal lobe, is where the visual stimuli are judged against their relationship with other objects three-dimensionally, giving the viewer the object's spatial location.

These two pathways work simultaneously to process the visual sensory information so that we know what we are seeing and also know its exact location, which is essential for our survival.

THE VISUAL–SENSORY SYSTEM

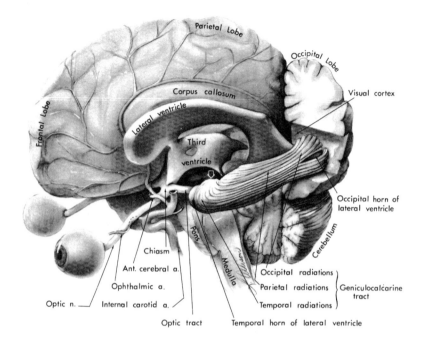

The left cerebral hemisphere has been removed.

Note the relationship of the optic nerve to the internal carotid and anterior communicating arteries.

Note the location of the parietal lobe (the "where" pathway). The temporal lobe (the "what" pathway) is not displayed here in order to show the structures between the two cerebral hemispheres.

THE VISUAL PATHWAY

Here are some examples of how things can go wrong when any part of the visual pathway is interrupted.

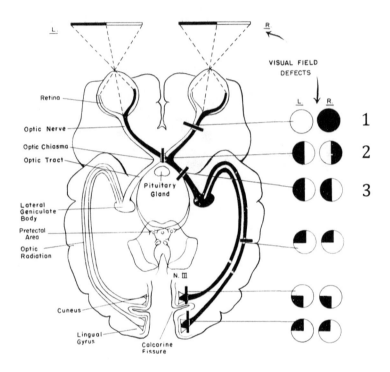

1. If the right optic nerve is damaged, such as severed in an injury, the eye becomes blind. The nerve can also be damaged by stroke or a tumor.

2. In the case of a pituitary gland tumor or craniopharyngioma near the midline behind the chiasm, the decussating fibers of the optic nerve are damaged and the visual impulses of the nasal halves of each retina are blocked, resulting in a **bitemporal hemianopia**. (The left eye does not perceive images in the left half of

its visual field, and the right eye does not perceive images in the right half of its visual field.)

3. If the right optic tract were destroyed, it would result in loss of function in the right halves of both retinas, with corresponding blindness in the left half of each visual field. This is called **left homonymous hemianopia**.

Cortical Blindness

This is an extremely rare condition in which extensive bilateral damage has been done to the cerebral visual pathways resulting in complete loss of vision. Patients with this condition have normal pupillary reactions because of the different pathways serving the pupillary light reflex and those carrying visual information. Examination of the fundus is normal.

Aneurysm

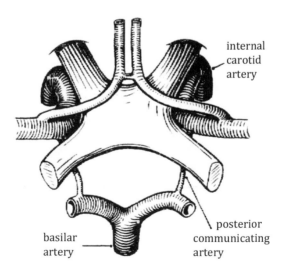

The optic chiasma lies within the circle of Willis.

Aneurysms commonly arise from this arterial circle and cause field defects by compressing the optic nerves, optic chiasma or optic tracts.

Tumor

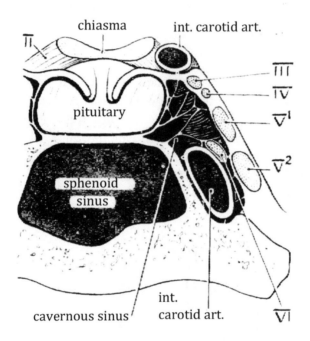

The pituitary gland sits behind the optic chiasma. A tumor may cause ischemia by squeezing small nutrient arteries, or edema and congestion by constricting the veins.

There are numerous other examples of visual field defects. Sometimes when the destruction of the tissue is incomplete, patients can have unusual visual fields.

Before MRI and CT scans were commonplace and accurate, the clinician often had to depend on the visual fields and other neurological findings to localize a lesion. Some neuro-ophthalmologists became very famous because they were so good at localizing the lesions.

Fewer ophthalmologists now go into the field of neuro-ophthalmology because such expertise is not as crucial as it used to be, as machines can do an excellent job localizing lesions in the brain and around the eye.

DIPLOPIA (Also read the pediatric chapter on the treatment of diplopia.)

Diplopia, or double vision, is a common complaint in medical practice and may be monocular or binocular.

Binocular double vision occurs when the images of the two eyes do not coincide so that the images produced are misaligned relative to one another. It disappears when one eye is covered. Cranial nerve palsies are the most common cause, with many of these cases brought on by diabetes mellitus and/or hypertension.

Monocular double vision is uncommon. It affects one eye only and can be caused by abnormalities of the lens, cornea or retina, resulting in splitting of the image.

Muscle disorders that can be accompanied by double vision include myasthenia gravis, Graves' disease and myotonic dystrophy.

Nerve problems associated with diplopia include conditions that affect the cranial nerves #3, #4 and #6 controlling the eye muscles. These conditions include diabetes mellitus, hypertension, multiple sclerosis and Guillain-Barre syndrome, with the first two being the most common.

Brain problems that can bring on double vision include vascular conditions such as strokes or aneurysms, or a tumor in the orbit or skull. Raised intracranial pressure can affect cranial nerve #6 (abducent) as it has the longest intracranial course. It may also be a side effect of some drugs such as ketamine, opioids and phenytoin.

STRABISMUS

In medical school, I used the formula LR6SO4 to remember how the six external ocular muscles are innervated.

The lateral rectus is supplied by nerve #6 (abducent), i.e. abduction (causing the eye to turn out), which is represented by LR6.

The superior oblique is supplied by nerve #4 (trochlear) which is represented by SO4.

The other four external muscles (the superior rectus, inferior rectus, medial rectus and inferior oblique), the internal muscles and the eyelid are supplied by the nerve #3 (oculomotor).

By remembering just #6 and #4, i.e., LR6SO4, I knew that the rest are innervated by nerve #3.

The four recti muscles pull directly on the eyeball so that they move in the direction of their names: superior, inferior, lateral and medial.

The oblique muscles move the eye outwards as well as up and down. Each muscle hooks around a "pulley" so that it moves the eye the opposite direction to which its name implies. The superior oblique muscle moves the eye down and out. The inferior oblique muscle moves it up and out.

Paralysis of a muscle means that the eye does not move fully in the direction in which it pulls. The eye therefore deviates in the opposite direction from the pull of the affected muscles.

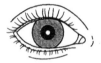 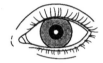

Primary position
Corneal light reflex is centrally (symmetrically) located in each eye.

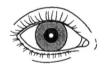 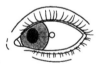

Left esotropia, i.e., the left eye is turned inward. This is because the left lateral rectus is weak and the eye is pulled in by the medial rectus. Cranial nerve #6 of the left side is affected. The most common cause of 6th nerve palsy is diabetes mellitus. Because of its long course, the 6th nerve palsy has no localizing value.
Which gaze makes the diplopia worse?

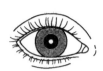 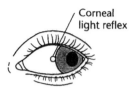

Corneal light reflex

Left exotropia, i.e., the left eye is turned outward. The medial rectus is weak and the eye is pulled out by the lateral rectus. The medial rectus is innervated by a branch of cranial nerve #3. If the pupil is not involved, it is likely to be of vascular origin such as diabetes, rather than a space occupying lesion in the brain.
Which gaze makes the diplopia worse?

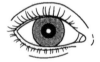 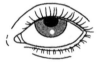

Left hypertropia, i.e., the left eye is turned upward. The inferior rectus is weak and the eye is pulled upward by the superior rectus. The inferior rectus is innervated by a branch of the cranial nerve #3. If the pupil is not involved, this too is most likely vascular in origin.
Which gaze makes the diplopia worse?

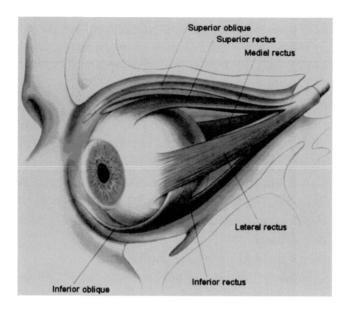

Superior oblique
Superior rectus
Medial rectus
Lateral rectus
Inferior rectus
Inferior oblique

If the left lateral rectus is paralyzed it cannot abduct, i.e., move the eye horizontally away from the nose.

The left medial rectus contracts unopposed and adduction occurs, i.e., the eye moves horizontally toward the nose, resulting in left esotropia as shown in the second drawing on page 99.

Cranial nerve #3, with its many branches, is a very important nerve and should be discussed further here. The intrinsic eye muscles are innervated by the autonomic systems and include the iris sphincter (constriction of the pupil) and the ciliary muscle (controls the accommodation of the lens), which are both innervated by the parasympathetic component of cranial nerve #3. The radial pupillodilator muscles (dilation of the pupil) are innervated by the ascending cervical sympathetic system. This information will be useful at the end of the chapter when neurological pupil disorders are discussed.

Since this chapter is on neuro-ophthalmology, I would like to go over what should be included in such an examination. Much of the neuro-ophthalmology examination is to evaluate cranial nerve #3.

Examination/Signs:
- Check for ptosis (drooping eyelid) to identify the affected side. Eyelid elevation is partly controlled by cranial nerve #3 (oculomotor nerve).
- Check the pupils to see if both are equal and react to light. The pupil is also controlled by cranial nerve #3.
- Pupil abnormalities may indicate the problem is intracranial.
- Check the optic nerve for papilledema.
- Identify which eye is affected and which direction of gaze is limited.

Fourth Nerve (Superior Oblique) Palsy is rare.

Symptoms include binocular vertical or oblique diplopia, difficulty reading and a sensation that objects appear tilted. If it is mild, it may be asymptomatic.

It is difficult to evaluate fourth nerve palsy and the list of differential diagnoses is long.

Sixth Nerve (Abducens) Palsy

The intracranial course of the abducens nerve (#6) is long, which means that it is prone to damage at many sites. Therefore, it has minimal localizing value. Isolated #6 nerve palsy is relatively common, especially in patients with diabetes.

In children, secondary strabismus may follow trauma to one or both eyes. Opacity of the media such as corneal scars or cataracts can cause the eye(s) of a child to deviate. A scar in the macula can also cause strabismus in a child.

In adults, secondary strabismus may be due to cranial nerve palsy from any of the following:

- Brain injury
- Intracranial mass such as brain tumor or abscess
- Stroke
- Diabetes mellitus
- Systemic hypertension
- Heart disease

In patients with recent onset of strabismus, a neurologist should be consulted.

Fifth Nerve (Trigeminal) Palsy

This nerve transmits sensation from the eye, particularly pain and touch from the cornea. The blink reflex prevents the cornea from being damaged. Damage to this nerve may result in corneal erosions from exposure and drying.

Herpes zoster may affect this nerve. When the ophthalmic division of the fifth nerve is involved, the patient develops a typical herpetic vesicular rash affecting the eyelids and forehead to the midline.

Seventh Nerve (Facial) Palsy

Symptoms: weakness or paralysis of one side of the face, excessive drooling and inability to close the eye.

The most common cause is Bell's palsy, which is idiopathic. Almost 90% of patients with Bell's palsy recover completely with observation alone within 2 months. Other causes of facial nerve palsy should be ruled out. The list is long and includes neoplasm, stroke, infections and neurological diseases.

The primary ocular complication is corneal exposure, which can be treated with artificial tears, lubricating ointment and taping of the eyelids.

PAPILLEDEMA

This is a term used to describe passive disc swelling associated with increased intracranial pressure. It is often used to suggest the association of brain tumor. This term is intended to prevent communicative confusion when other forms of disc swelling are considered.

Some other causes of "swollen" disc:
Metabolic: proliferative retinopathies, etc.
Inflammatory: papillitis, neuroretinitis
Systemic Disease: anemia, hypoxia, hypertension
Vascular: ischemic neuropathy, cranial arteritis
Infiltrative: lymphoma
Ocular Disease: uveitis, vein occlusion
Elevated Intracranial Pressure: mass lesion, pseudotumor cerebri, and hydrocephalus.

Clinical Characteristics of Papilledema and Optic Neuritis

Papilledema:
- No visual loss
- No eye pain
- Always bilateral
- No abnormality of pupil
- Normal visual acuity
- Variable degree of disc swelling and hemorrhages
- Visual prognosis is good after relief of intracranial pressure

Optic Neuritis:
- Loss of central vision
- Tender globe, pain on motion
- Can be in one or both eyes
- Diminished light reaction on side of neuritis
- Variable degree of disc swelling
- Vision usually returns to normal or functional levels

GRADE III PAPILLEDEMA

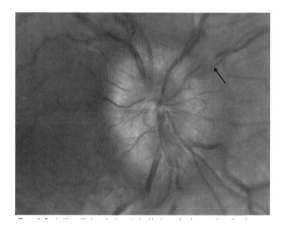

- Blurring of disc margin
- Hyperemia of the disc
- Obscuration of the wall of vessels crossing disc margin
- Elevation of disc
- Hemorrhages on or near disc
- Spontaneous venous pulsations in some patients

Idiopathic Intracranial Hypertension (IIH):

This condition is also known as Pseudotumor Cerebri. IIH is a condition of unknown cause characterized by elevated cerebrospinal fluid (CSF) pressure and papilledema. It is most commonly found in obese women of childbearing age.

The main symptoms are headache, transient visual obscuration, blurred vision and horizontal diplopia. Visual loss caused by disc swelling is the major permanent sequel of IIH.

Diagnosis is by elimination of other causes of elevated CSF pressure such as viral, bacterial and fungal infections, tumors, and inflammatory or metabolic conditions.

Use of vitamin A or multivitamins in high doses may be associated with this condition.

Treatment with a carbonic anhydrase inhibitor such as acetazolamide (Diamox) has been generally effective.

AMAUROSIS FUGAX

Amaurosis Fugax (*fleeting darkness* in Greek) is not an uncommon complaint in a primary care provider's office. It is always vascular in origin.

If the partial blindness is transient, it may be caused by retinal arteriolar spasm. When the blindness is permanent, it is caused by blockage of the retinal arteries by cholesterol plaque.

If the cholesterol plaque leads to Central Retinal Artery Occlusion, examination will show a "cherry-red spot" in the center of the macula.

If the problem is systemic, it may be associated with:
- Carotid artery stenosis
- Malignant hypertension
- Patients with long history of heavy smoking

- Vascular insufficiency of the vertebral-basilar arterial system
- Preceding a cerebrovascular accident

Treatment:
If the loss of vision is caused by a blockage of the central retinal artery by a cholesterol embolus (Hollenhorst plaque), and the blockage is less than half an hour in duration, the patient should be asked to breathe into a bag, in the hope that increasing the concentration of carbon dioxide in the bloodstream will cause dilation of the artery and allow the embolus to flow away from the center, thus sparing the macula (central vision). Massaging the eye may also sometimes dislodge the plaque. If these non-invasive methods do not work, then a more drastic procedure may be needed.

Paracentesis (removal of fluid from the anterior chamber of the eye—the space between the cornea and iris) is the last resort. This is done using a #30 gauge (short) needle attached to a small plastic syringe. Only topical anesthesia is required. After going through the cornea, withdraw 0.2 ml of aqueous fluid. This should be done under sterile conditions and with good visualization with the loupe or slit lamp.

Permanent blindness occurs after 90 minutes if the plaque is not dislodged.

I am not advocating that primary care providers do paracentesis. However, I think it is important to be aware of what procedure is available in the unlikely event that the primary care provider is presented a patient with such a problem and no help is within reach. During my internship, I determined that should I be presented with a patient who was dying from a subdural hematoma, and I was in a remote area without any surgeon nearby, I was willing to do a burr hole surgery to save the patient's life even though I was not a neurosurgeon. (I had assisted in several such surgeries.) It is important to always be aware and prepared.

TEMPORAL ARTERITIS

Also known as giant cell arteritis or cranial arteritis, temporal arteritis is a systemic vasculitis of unknown cause that can lead to blindness, stroke and death. It typically occurs in patients aged 60 years or older, and symptoms include pain on chewing, headache, temporal artery tenderness or scalp tenderness. Anorexia, weight loss, fever, malaise or depression may be associated. Elevated ESR is associated with most cases.

Diagnosis is made by positive biopsy of the temporal artery, but a normal temporal artery biopsy does not rule it out. If untreated, it can lead to blindness and death. This condition should always be considered if an elderly patient comes in with headache and visual loss. Treatment is with large doses of corticosteroids.

MIGRAINE

The throbbing headache of a migraine is usually unilateral. It is often associated with nausea and preceded by visual disturbances and other symptoms. The visual aura is often described as wave-like rippling, which is believed to be caused by vasoconstriction followed by a phase of vasodilation. The headache phase is believed to be caused by the edema of the arterial wall. This condition must be distinguished from other more serious conditions such as ischemic attacks.

Treatments include propranolol (a beta-adrenergic blocker) and other more standard drugs such as antidepressants, analgesics and sedatives. Use of ergot derivatives (vasoconstrictors) for prophylaxis must be done with great caution, as it may worsen the neurologic deficit. A serotonin agonist, Sumatriptan, acts as a select cerebral vasoconstrictor and has been effective in treating migraine.

NEUROLOGICAL PUPIL DISORDERS

Horner's Syndrome

This rare syndrome results from an interruption of the sympathetic nerve supply to the eye and is characterized by the classic triad of miosis (constricted pupil), partial ptosis (drooping eyelid) and loss of hemi-facial sweating (anhidrosis).

Causes include brainstem stroke or tumor, tumor or infection of the lung apex, and carotid artery ischemia.

Adie's Tonic Pupil

Here, the parasympathetic (constrictor) pathway is damaged on its way to the iris sphincter muscles. The pupil is dilated and does not constrict to light. The pupil will constrict slowly to near vision. Unlike Horner's Syndrome, the potential causes for damage to the parasympathetic pathway are usually more benign such as a viral infection.

Argyll Robertson Pupil

This condition refers to a form of light-near dissociation in which the pupils are small and respond poorly to light but promptly to near vision testing. Both pupils are always involved and respond poorly to dilating agents. This abnormality is probably due to a lesion in the light reflex path of the midbrain.

It has been seen in patients with diabetes, but it is generally associated with neurosyphilis and workup for such should be initiated with the patient.

I am not suggesting that the busy primary care provider evaluate every abnormal pupil. It is important to be aware of such abnormalities and take the entire clinical picture into consideration as to what should be done.

CHAPTER 11: PEDIATRIC OPHTHALMOLOGY AND STRABISMUS

Like many medical fields, the examination and treatment of children is often more difficult than it is with adults. In some situations, such as a corneal foreign body, the child may need to be restrained in order to perform an adequate examination or to provide the necessary treatment.

EXAMINATION:

Visual acuity testing may or may not be necessary or possible.

Check eyelids for ptosis.

Check pupils for symmetry and response to light. A white pupil (leukocoria) may indicate a serious problem such as retinoblastoma or cataract.

Check cornea for size and clarity. A cloudy, enlarged cornea and tearing may indicate infantile glaucoma.

Photophobia may indicate keratitis (herpes simplex), uveitis or infantile glaucoma.

Check eyes for deviation. The eye with the deviation should be assumed to have an organic lesion such as retinoblastoma or toxoplasmosis involving the macula until proven otherwise. Strabismus is common in childhood. Untreated, the child can develop amblyopia (lazy eye).

Check for nystagmus (involuntary eye movement). If present, it would indicate poor visual acuity caused by disorders such as macular scars, macular hypoplasia or optic nerve hypoplasia. There are also other causes for nystagmus.

Look for the red reflex as described in Chapter 2. Absence of a red reflex may suggest the presence of cataract, retinoblastoma, ROP (retinopathy of prematurity) or vitreous opacity.

Check the optic nerve and retina if possible. Method of examination is described in Chapter 2.

Ophthalmic ointment generally works better than drops for children.

Shaken Baby Syndrome

When a baby presents with retinal hemorrhages, abuse should be ruled out. The hemorrhages can be caused by violent shaking, choking or direct eye or head trauma. Papilledema and vitreous hemorrhage may occur in association, along with subdural or subarachnoid hemorrhage or cerebral contusion.

It is required by law in many countries to report suspected abuse to the authorities. Good documentation of the findings is essential.

Retinopathy of Prematurity (ROP)

The formation of the retinal vasculature begins at about week 16 of gestation from the optic disc outwards. This vasculature reaches the nasal retinal-edge at about 36 weeks. If a baby is born premature, there are areas in the peripheral retina that have not yet developed a good blood supply and can become ischemic, which can produce VEGF, which in turn promotes neovascularization. These new vessels can bleed and can eventually cause retinal detachment.

If neovascularization is detected, it can be treated with laser or cryotherapy to prevent such a complication. Anti-VEGF drugs are also being used to stop neovascularization.

Examination of the premature infant for ROP is difficult and should be done by a retinal specialist.

Strabismus

Paralytic strabismus usually occurs in older people, with diplopia being a common complaint. Good vision is usually found in both eyes. Neurologic work-up is usually required.

Non-paralytic strabismus usually occurs in infants and children. Diplopia rarely occurs because the child suppresses the deviated eye, which is often amblyopic. Ophthalmic work-up is required.

Common causes of **neural paralytic strabismus** (Cranial nerves #3, #4 and #6):

In patients younger than 40, the causes are congenital defects, head trauma, cranial artery aneurysms, multiple sclerosis and others.

In patients over 40, the causes are diabetes, cerebral vascular accident and others.

When the paralysis is in the muscle, it can occur at any age. Some of the causes are: myasthenia gravis, hyperthyroidism, blowout fractures, and muscular injuries.

Esotropia (ET) means deviation of one eye nasally.
Exotropia (XT) means deviation of one eye outward.
Hypertropia (HT) means deviation of one eye upward.
Hypotropia (HoT) means deviation of one eye downward.

Ocular deviations are measured in prism diopters. When light passes through a prism, it is bent toward the base of the prism. The prism diopter is not the same as the lens diopter, which measures myopia or hyperopia.

Diplopia can be corrected with prisms. This is usually done for patients whose diplopia is caused by diabetes or strokes and will improve with time. Prism is usually a temporary treatment. Diplopia can also be relieved by patching one eye. Botulinum toxin (Botox) can be injected into one of the muscles to treat diplopia temporarily.

PRISMS

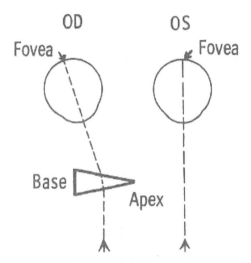

In this patient with a right esotropia, the right fovea is turned temporally. In order to focus the light on the right fovea, a prism (with the apex nasally) is placed in front of the right eye, eliminating the diplopia.

If the patient had an exotropia, the apex would be pointed temporally, i.e., the prism apex always points in the direction of the deviation.

Fresnel Prisms

These are thin, transparent sheets of plastic. One side sticks to the patient's glasses and the other side has special grooves in it that create a prism effect, changing the way light enters the eye. As the deviation lessens with time, the amount of prisms can also be reduced, making this a simple, safe and effective treatment for diplopia.

When the deviation is felt to be permanent, surgery on the muscles can be considered. Each eye muscle can be weakened, strengthened or moved.

Strabismus Surgery

Strabismus is treated surgically early in the US, which explains why we hardly see any children with this condition anymore. Until I went into ophthalmology, it was a mystery to me how the surgeon could get to the muscles!

RECTI

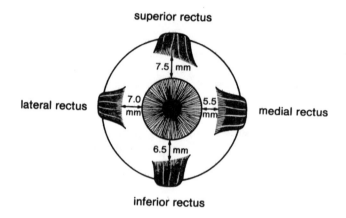

LEFT EYE

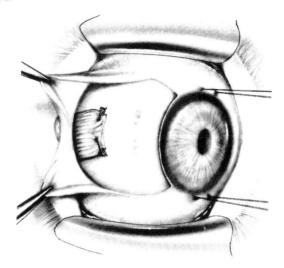

Resection of the left medial rectus muscles. The muscle is reattached about 5 mm behind the original insertion, essentially making it about 5 mm longer.

RIGHT EYE

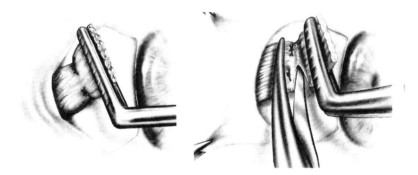

Resection of the right lateral rectus muscle. The muscle is detached from the original insertion. A 5 mm segment is cut and reattached to the original insertion, essentially making it about 5 mm shorter.

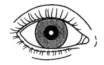 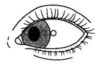

Left esotropia

Which muscle needs to be recessed and which one should be resected in the left eye?

(Lateral rectus resection and medial rectus recession)

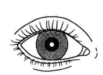 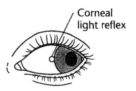

Corneal light reflex

Left exotropia

Which muscle needs to be recessed and which one should be resected in the left eye?

(Medial rectus resection and lateral rectus recession)

Amblyopia (lazy eye)

Amblyopia is decreased vision in an eye from disuse during childhood development. The visual pathway is plastic during childhood until around 6 to 9 years of age. During the plastic phase, the connections between the retina and visual cortex are still developing. An image sent from the eye to the visual cortex has to be clear in order for the child to learn to see. If the eye has a severe refractive error, is misaligned, or has a cataract or anything that prevents a clear image from forming, it could lead to permanent visual loss that can't be corrected. This is the reason why a baby with congenital cataract must have surgery early on.

With a misaligned eye, the child simply ignores that eye, and it can become amblyopic. This is why the "normal" eye is sometimes patched: to force the child to use the misaligned eye and prevent amblyopia. Sometimes parents don't understand why the ophthalmologist patches the child's good eye!

Retinoblastoma

This is a tumor of the primitive retinal photoreceptors that grows on the retina, forming a white mass that can completely fill the eye. It is the most common primary malignant ocular tumor in children, but it is very rare, with less than 500 new cases reported each year in the US. If undetected, it could result in the death of a child. The tumor spreads by growing down the optic nerve toward the brain. If detected early, the overall survival rate in the US is about 90%.

CHAPTER 12: OCULAR MANIFESTATIONS OF SYSTEMIC DISEASES

Ocular conditions can arise secondary to systemic disease, and knowing their connection will often help with diagnosis. The first section below discusses the most common conditions, followed by a list of less commonly encountered conditions. The third section covers ocular side effects or adverse reactions to various drugs.

MORE COMMON DISEASES WITH OCULAR MANIFESTATIONS

AIDS:
"Cotton wool" spots on retina; uveitis; candida chorioretinitis; cytomegalovirus (CMV) retinitis; keratitis; herpes zoster; Kaposi's sarcoma of eyelids and conjunctiva.

AIDS used to be a fatal disease and the complications listed used to be seen worldwide. In most developed countries these complications are now much less common because most HIV patients are adequately treated. But in some underdeveloped countries, these complications still exist because patients are often inadequately treated or not treated at all.

Hypertensive Retinopathy:
In the less severe form, the vessels show attenuation and increased light reflex, the reddish brown of the so-called "copper wire" reflex. Focal and diffuse constriction and AV crossing phenomena (nicking) may be noted.

In the more severe form, retinal edema, hemorrhages, and cotton-wool spots are present. The optic disc may show edema, which can be mistaken for papilledema. But the disc edema in severe hypertension is due to infarction and hypoxia of the optic disc itself. (The term papilledema is reserved for disc edema associated with elevated cerebrospinal fluid pressures.)

A prolonged hypertensive state may result in the formation of a macular star of hard exudates, which can permanently damage the central vision. The presence of hard exudates in the macula suggests that these patients may also have involvement of the kidney and other organs.

Lupus erythematous:
Retinal vasculitis is a complication associated with lupus. The inflammation in the vessels causes leakage in the vessel walls, macular edema, and all the other signs associated with ischemic response of the retina.

Toxoplasmosis, Crohn's inflammatory bowel disease, multiple sclerosis, sarcoidosis, syphilis and Eales Disease are also associated with retinal vasculitis.

Lyme disease:
Caused by the spirochete Borrelia burgdorferi, Lyme disease is an immune-mediated inflammatory disease with numerous ocular, neuro-ophthalmic, and systemic manifestations.

Eye findings may include optic neuritis, papilledema, pseudo-tumor cerebri, diplopia secondary to third and sixth nerve atrophy, and Bell's palsy. Other eye manifestations may include retinal hemorrhages, exudative retinal detachments and iritis. Treatment is controversial and beyond the scope of this book.

Sickle-cell disease or sickle-cell anemia:
This disease may lead to various acute and chronic complications throughout the body, several of which have a high mortality rate. It is caused by sickle-shaped red blood cells that obstruct capillaries and restrict blood flow to an organ, resulting in ischemia.

The complication in the eye is retinal neovascularization, which is most common at about the equator plane supra-temporally. This area is very difficult to see with the direct ophthalmoscope. The complication of neovascularization is vitreous hemorrhage. If allowed to proliferate, it can cause traction retinal detachment.

The treatment is laser photocoagulation to the areas of neovascularization.

LESS COMMON SYSTEMIC DISEASES WHICH MAY BE ASSOCIATED WITH OCULAR CONDITIONS

Albinism:
Nystagmus; poor vision secondary to poor macular development and refractive error; choroidal vessels visible with the ophthalmoscope because of hypopigmentation of RPE; light sensitivity because of light iris

Anemia:
Conjunctiva appears pale. In severe cases retinal hemorrhages may be present.

Atopic Dermatitis:
Cataracts and keratoconus

Cystic Fibrosis:
Papilledema and retinal hemorrhages

Down's Syndrome (Trisomy 21):
The typical up-slanted palpebral fissures; cataract; myopia; strabismus; amblyopia; degenerative changes in the cornea sometimes leading to keratoconus; glaucoma and retinovascular anomalies

Galactosemia:
Cataract

Glomerulonephritis:
Hypertensive retinopathy

Gout:
Uveitis; episcleritis

Herpes Zoster:
Uveitis; keratitis; dermatitis of the ophthalmic branch of the 5th cranial nerve

Hyperthyroidism:
Proptosis (protrusion of the eyeball); papilledema

Lead Poisoning:
Papilledema; optic atrophy

Migraine:
Eye pain; transient visual disturbance (e.g., flashing lights, hemianopia, waves); small pupil

Multiple Sclerosis:
Retrobulbar (behind the eyeball) optic neuritis; optic atrophy; diplopia

Myasthenia Gravis:
Extraocular muscle weakness; ptosis

Neurofibromatosis:
Optic gliomas (usually slow-growing and non-cancerous); orbital and lid tumors

Niacin deficiency (pellagra):
Optic neuritis

Polycythemia:
Papilledema; dilated retinal veins

Rheumatoid Arthritis:
Thinning of the sclera; uveitis

Rubella (congenital):
Cataract; uveitis; retinopathy

Sarcoid:
Uveitis; perivenous infiltrates in retina

Sjogren's Syndrome:
Dry eyes; corneal erosions

Syphilis:
Uveitis; optic neuritis; cataracts; lens dislocation; chorioretinitis (inflammation of choroid and retina); Argyll Robertson pupil

Temporal Arteritis:
Severe vasculitis affecting the optic nerve, leading to transient or permanent visual loss

Thiamine deficiency (beriberi):
Optic neuritis; weakness of the extraocular muscles

Toxemia:
Hypertensive retinopathy

Toxoplasmosis:
Chorioretinitis

Tuberculosis:
Uveitis; chorioretinitis

Tuberous Sclerosis:
Retinal tumors

Vitamin C deficiency (scurvy):
Hemorrhages of the eye—inside and outside.

Vitamin D Deficiency:
Papilledema; cataract

Von Hippel-Lindau Disease:
Retinal hemangiomas

Wilson's Disease:
Kayser-Fleischer ring (copper deposits in the peripheral cornea); cataract secondary to copper deposits in the lens

DRUGS TOXICITY:

Amiodarone:
Pigment whorl on cornea

Chloramphenicol:
Optic neuritis

Chloroquine/Hydroxychloroquine toxicity:
These are used in the long-term treatment of lupus erythematosus and rheumatoid arthritis. A total dose of 100-300g or more of chloroquine can lead to a toxic effect on the macula at the RPE. Hydroxychloroquine can be tolerated better.

The earliest functional changes are decreased sensitivity to the red-green on the Ishihara color test. The so-called "bull's eye" maculopathy can be detected by fluorescein angiography.

Chlorpromazine (Thorazine):
Pigmentary retinopathy; blurred vision

Contraceptive Hormones:
Central vein occlusion; optic neuritis; migraine

Digitalis:
Yellow vision

Ethambutol:
Decreased color vision and visual acuity secondary to retrobulbar optic neuritis

Haloperidol (Haldol):
Blurred vision; oculogyric crises (prolonged involuntary upward deviation)

Steroids:
Both topical and systemic steroids can cause cataract and glaucoma; papilledema from systemic steroids

Tamsulosin (Flomax):
Floppy iris syndrome—may cause complications during cataract surgery

Tetracycline:
Papilledema

Thioridazine (Mellaril):
Pigmentary retinopathy

Topiramate(Topomax)—Anti-convulsive:
May cause angle closure glaucoma

Viagra (sildenafil), Cialis (tadalifil) and Levitra (vardenafil):
Some patients may experience transient, mild impairment of color discrimination, which has been described as a blue-colored tinge of vision. No long-term effects can be identified so far. There have been a few cases of ischemic optic neuropathy and central serous retinopathy reported, but the association has not been confirmed.

Vitamin A Intoxication:
Papilledema

Vitamin D Intoxication:
Band keratopathy

CHAPTER 13: EYE DISEASES IN DEVELOPING COUNTRIES

In some developing countries, eye conditions that are no longer seen in more developed countries are still prevalent, and sometimes in advanced stages. The main problem is poverty, which often leads to poor and unhygienic living conditions (no water or bathroom in many cases), lack of education, malnutrition, and poor infrastructure with inadequate medical care.

This chapter helps health care providers in developing countries understand what they should look for, and helps volunteer health care providers from developed countries be aware of what they may encounter.

TRACHOMA

Trachoma is a contagious bacterial (Chlamydia) infection of the eye. If left untreated, repeated trachoma infection can cause severe scarring of the inside of the eyelid and can cause the eyelashes to scratch the cornea (trichiasis). In addition to causing pain, trichiasis permanently damages the cornea and can lead to irreversible blindness. Almost 8 million people are visually impaired by this disease; 500 million are at risk of blindness throughout 57 endemic countries.

The World Health Organization has targeted trachoma for elimination by 2020 through a public health strategy known as S.A.F.E.:

- Surgery to correct trichiasis;
- Antibiotics to treat active infection;
- Facial cleanliness; and
- Environmental improvements in endemic areas to reduce disease transmission.

Trachoma is spread from person to person and from eye to eye by poor hygiene and contaminated fingers. Houseflies are implicated as they seek the moisture of mucous membranes (the conjunctiva).

Diagnosis:
Examination can be done with a loupe and flashlight. Check for inturned eyelashes and corneal opacity. Examine the inside of the upper eyelid for follicles, inflammation or scarring. The patient may complain of pain or itching, or, if scarring has occurred, a feeling of sand behind the eyelids.

Treatment:
Tetracycline 1% ointment is very effective. Topical erythromycin may be substituted if topical tetracycline is not available.

Oral tetracycline may be given against trachoma. Children and pregnant women are contraindicated. A one-time 1-gram dose of Azithromycin is also effective and seems to have few serious adverse side effects in children over 6 months of age.

Surgical management:
Surgery can be performed to correct the deformity of entropion and trichiasis to prevent further damage to the cornea. The goal is to keep the disease from progressing to this stage.

VITAMIN A DEFICIENCY

Vitamin A is needed for the growth and functioning of surface tissues, which include the skin's epithelium and the mucous membranes, and of ocular tissues, especially the cornea and retina.

Keratomalacia (softening and melting of the cornea) is the most severe form of vitamin A deficiency.

In my book, Silk Road on My Mind, *I describe an infant I examined in Xinjiang (northwest China). She was from a remote area of the province and was seen at the hospital with multiple problems, one of which was melting of her cornea due to vitamin A deficiency.*

Even mild vitamin A deficiency can reduce the chances of survival in early childhood. Chronic vitamin A deficiency can cause night blindness.

Treatment and Prevention:
Alleviation of poverty is the main prevention. Vitamin A occurs in eggs, milk, liver and fish. It also occurs in the precursor form in dark green leafy and yellow vegetables, tubers and fruits.
Vitamin A capsules (200,000 IU) are inexpensive and available almost anywhere.

ONCHOCERCIASIS (RIVER BLINDNESS)

This is a chronic parasitic infection that can cause damage inside the eye from uveitis, and blindness by scarring the cornea and retina. Over 100 million people are at risk of infection in Africa and a few small areas in South America and Yemen.

Onchocerciasis is caused by a filarial nematode worm, Onchocerca volvulus. It is transmitted by the bite of a black fly, which breeds in fast-flowing rivers. Mircrofilarial prelarvae occur in human skin, which are ingested by the female black fly and transmitted to another human host when she bites. The larvae then develop into adult worms in the skin, forming nodules. The microfilariae can migrate throughout the body and can be found in the bloodstream, and are found in high concentration in the eye. The parasite causes blindness by damaging and scarring in the cornea, retina, choroid, and optic nerve.

Patients with active infection of the parasite suffer greatly with eye pain and loss of vision as well as pain caused by the skin nodules. Diagnosis can be made from a skin biopsy.

Medical Management:
Ivermectin (Mectizan), a broad-spectrum anti-parasitic drug is safe and has been successful in treatment of the disease, but it only kills the larvae, not the adult worms.

A clinical trial of a new drug called Moxidectin, which not only kills the larvae but also sterilizes the adult worms, has been launched. If successful, it could eliminate this dreadful disease that has plagued so many countries for centuries.

Management of Ocular Onchocerciasis:
Management of the active disease involves controlling the keratitis, chorioretinitis and uveitis. The damage done cannot be reversed.

Prevention:
- Reduce the number of infected individuals through treatment.
- Interrupt the transmission by controlling the Simulium black fly.

LOA LOA (LOIASIS) OR AFRICAN EYE WORM

This disease is caused by the nematode (round worm) Loa loa. It is spread by repeated bites from deerflies in West and Central Africa. The adult worms live between layers of connective tissue. It is most dramatic when a worm can be seen moving underneath the conjunctiva or inside the eye. *(If you are interested, check YouTube for video of surgical removal of the worm.)* It looks scary, but the worm usually does little damage to the eye, unlike onchocerciasis, which often leads to blindness.

Local people typically don't get loiasis as severely as visitors do. Most people with the infection do not have any symptoms.

There are areas where onchocerciasis and loiasis are co-endemic. This has complicated the attempt to eradicate onchocerciasis, because if Ivermectin is given to a patient with a heavy Loa loa worm infection in the brain, it can cause coma or even death due to the severe inflammation that occurs when the worms die.

HANSEN'S DISEASE (LEPROSY)

In medical school I did a research paper on some patients with Hansen's disease and used the term "leprosy." The professor advised me never to use the word again because it carries such stigma, and to say Hansen's disease instead.

Hansen's disease is caused by mycobacterium leprae. It is a chronic disease that affects the skin, peripheral nerves, and extremities. When it involves the face and nerves of the face, the eyes cannot close completely, leading to exposure keratitis with corneal scarring. It can also cause uveitis and secondary glaucoma. Blindness may result. Ocular complications can be prevented by early detection of the disease.

Patients with this condition can be ostracized by their own communities because of their appearance and fear of contracting the disease. It is transmitted by prolonged exposure to those infected with the mycobacterium.

This disease is found in several regions: sub-Saharan Africa, the Middle East, the Indian subcontinent, Indochina and islands of the Western Pacific. (*In 2014, on a medical mission to Western Samoa, I examined some patients with Hansen's disease for eye complications.*)

Corneal opacity can occur if the mycobacterium leprae invade the cornea along the pathway of the corneal nerves, making it insensitive. Without sensation, corneal injuries are not noted, leading to corneal erosion, ulceration, and scarring.

Medical treatment involves long-term multidrug therapy with Dirampicin once monthly, Clofazimine once monthly and a maintenance dose daily, and Dapsone daily.

Patients with Hansen's disease are usually under the care of providers with specialized training in this area to coordinate the difficult management of multiple problems, especially those involving the eye.

EBOLA VIRUS (EBOV)

Ebola is a small, single stranded RNA virus. The vector is the fruit bat. Large mammals including humans, apes, and pigs are susceptible. It is spread by direct contact with body fluids including saliva, vomit, urine, blood, feces, semen, and intra-ocular fluids.

The virus causes a severe hemorrhagic fever with hematemesis, bloody diarrhea, abdominal cramping, severe dehydration and death in over 80% of the cases within a few days. During the 2013-2015 epidemic in Western Africa, it primarily affected Sierra Leone, Liberia and Guinea. About 30,000 people were infected; many were health care workers. Survivors were shown to have the virus remaining in the semen and eyes (aqueous and vitreous).

Treatment (as of 2015) is primarily supportive, with intravenous therapy to treat dehydration, blood pressure support, and oxygenation. There is no known antiviral treatment. Some patients have been treated systemically with serum from infected surviving individuals, which contains antibodies effective against the Ebola virus.

Late ocular manifestations include uveitis, wherein patients present with blurred vision, eye pain, retinal hemorrhages and photophobia. About 40% of survivors have blinds spots in their visual fields.

Because the aqueous and vitreous may contain the virus in survivors, great care must be taken to avoid exposure to these fluids, such as when treating patients with penetrating trauma or those requiring eye surgery, including cataract surgery.

These diseases are also found in developed countries, but patients are more likely to be adequately treated and less likely to suffer from opportunistic infections.

AIDS
Associated retinopathies:
- Cytomegalovirus
- Pneumocystis carinii
- Syphilis
- Acute retinal necrosis (herpes zoster or herpes simplex)
- Toxoplasmosis
- Cryptococcus

SYPHILIS

It is especially important for primary care providers to know that this disease can affect the patient's eye. The infection occurs in phases. **Primary syphilis** is characterized by a chancre, an erythematous papule that evolves into a painless ulcer at the site of inoculation. If untreated, those with primary syphilis progress to secondary syphilis 4 to 10 weeks after the appearance of the chancre.

Secondary syphilis (untreated or inadequately treated) is known to cause retinitis that can lead to blindness. Usually there is evidence of anterior segment inflammation, such as cells in the anterior chamber. Lymphadenopathy and a maculopapular rash, which often presents on the palms and soles, typify secondary syphilis.

Tertiary syphilis may develop after a variable period of latency if untreated. The central nervous system may be involved. In tertiary syphilis, chorio-retinitis, neuro-retinitis and occlusive vascular disease may be observed.

The presence of ocular disease warrants treatment with IV penicillin for 10 to 14 days.

The diagnosis of syphilis necessitates testing for HIV, as co-infection is common due to similar risk factors. All patients with syphilitic retinitis should be presumed to also have neurosyphilis.

TOXOPLASMOSIS

This condition is spread by cat feces and is one of the most common causes of posterior uveitis worldwide. The parasite Toxoplasma gondii is another one of the many opportunistic infections often found in immunocompromised patients.

Standard treatment consists of pyrimethamine, sulfa drugs or clindamycin, or a combination.

TUBERCULOSIS

One third of the world's population has latent infection with mycobacterium tuberculosis. Only a very small portion of these individuals will manifest signs of the disease. In patients with tuberculosis, it is rare for the disease to involve the eye. When it does, it causes uveitis.

STRABISMUS IN CHILDREN

It is estimated that 2% of the world's population suffers from strabismus. In the US and other industrialized nations, patients with this condition are treated early. In developing countries, this is one of the leading causes of vision loss. Many of these individuals become societal outcasts and have difficulty finding spouses or jobs. Because it is not life-threatening or a danger to the sight, it is frequently low on the priority list for treatment.

More technicians should be trained to do this sort of surgery in developing countries.

COMMENTS ON EYE CARE IN DEVELOPING COUNTRIES

In addition to programs such as the World Health Organization's S.A.F.E. initiative mentioned at the beginning of the chapter, there are many other groups working on eye care issues around the world.

The Aravind Eye Hospitals is a hospital chain in India founded by Dr. G. Venkataswamy. It has grown into a network of eye hospitals and has had a major impact in eradicating cataract-related blindness in India and some other parts of the world. This model has been copied in other countries. The company produces its own intra-ocular lenses at a price of $2 each. At its Madurai, Tamil Nadu campus, it regularly trains surgeons and technicians from around the world, including some provinces in China.

Aravind is focused on efficiency and hygiene. It can do a cataract surgery with an IOL for as little as $35. Its infection rate is about 4/1000 in contrast to the international norm of 6/1000 surgeries.

The Fred Hollows Foundation was founded by Dr. Fred Hollows in 1992 and is based in Australia. The Foundation focuses on treating and preventing blindness all over the world (so far, over 19 countries), particularly in the Pacific, South and Southeast Asia and Africa. It also provides training for local eye care providers and has built hospitals in several countries. It has provided extensive training of medical staff and screening for poor vision and eye disease, and has subsidized treatment and provision of equipment and infrastructures in countries such as Eritrea, Kenya, Rwanda, South Africa, and Tanzania.

Orbis International is a non-profit organization dedicated to saving sight worldwide. It is well known for its "Flying Eye Hospital," an ophthalmic hospital and teaching facility located on board a jumbo jet. Its entire staff, including the pilot and flight crew, are volunteers. It has served in over 100 countries. Orbis is headquartered in New York with offices in Toronto, Dublin, Hong Kong, Macau, Shanghai, Taipei, and Cape Town. It now has a telemedicine program called Cybersight (http://www.cybersight.org), which uses the Internet to connect eye care professionals for one-on-one collaboration and mentoring.

The Hawaiian Eye Foundation, based in Honolulu, has made numerous expeditions to Pacific Basin countries to provide humanitarian eye surgery and training, including recent training programs in Vietnam and Myanmar to teach advanced techniques to eye surgeons. It also funds research projects and operates outreach programs that include training scholarships and donations of equipment and supplies.

These are just a few of the many organizations that provide eye services to different parts of the world. In some countries, because of the brain drain of professionals to wealthier countries, there are tremendous shortages of physicians, and ophthalmologists in particular. Some charity organizations have trained non-physician technicians to do eye surgeries. It seems that these pioneering programs have helped a large number of patients who would otherwise not have access to surgery.

When I was in Western Samoa in 2014, I was again reminded of the human and economic costs of blindness. *(I am referring to people who become blind late in life. Most blind people, just as with sighted people, lead very productive lives when they have access to education and opportunities.)* The daughter (a young school teacher) of a woman in her early fifties who had recently gone blind from diabetic retinopathy sadly told me that after her mother lost her sight, she had to quit her job to take care of her—at least until her mother could learn to get around and be left alone. When a person goes blind, it affects the whole family. This case was especially tragic because the woman's blindness could have been easily prevented through laser treatment.

Similarly, the thousands of patients affected by the complications of trachoma could have been spared their suffering by using a small tube of ointment costing less than a dollar!

The goal of this book is to educate both health care providers and patients so that they are aware of eye disorders and possible treatments and understand that in almost all cases, people do not have to go blind. Life is already a challenge for many in developing countries without preventable blindness adding to their difficulties.

GLOSSARY

Accommodation: The adjustment of the eye for seeing at different distances, by changing the shape of the lens via the action of the ciliary muscles, thus focusing a clear image on the retina.

Agnosia: Inability to recognize common things despite an intact visual apparatus.

Albinism: A hereditary deficiency of pigment in the retinal pigment epithelium, iris, and choroid.

Amaurosis fugax: Transient loss of vision.

Amblyopia: Reduced visual acuity that cannot be corrected with lenses, in the absence of detectable anatomic defect in the eye or visual pathways.

Aniridia: Absence of the iris.

Aniseikonia: When the image seen by one eye differs in size or shape from that seen by the other.

Anisometropia: Difference in refractive error of the eyes.

Anophthalmos: Absence of a true eyeball.

Anterior chamber: The space filled with aqueous bounded by the cornea anteriorly and by the iris posteriorly.

Aphakia: Absence of the lens.

Aqueous: Clear, watery fluid that fills the anterior and posterior chambers.

Asthenopia: Eye fatigue caused by tiring.

Astigmatism: Refractive error that prevents the light rays from coming to a single focus on the retina because of different degrees of refraction in the various meridians of the cornea.

Binocular vision: Ability of the eyes to focus on one object and fuse the two images into one.

Blepharitis: Inflammation of the eyelids.

Blepharoptosis: Drooping of the eyelid.

Blepharospasm: Involuntary spasm of the eyelids.

Blind spot: Blank area in the visual field, which corresponds to the light rays that come to a focus on the optic nerve.

Blindness: In the US, the usual definition of legal blindness is corrected visual acuity of 20/200 or less in the better eye, or a visual field of less than 20 degrees in the better eye.

Buphthalmos: Large eyeball in infantile glaucoma.

Canal of Schlemm: A circular modified venous structure in the anterior chamber angle.

Canaliculus: Small tear drainage tube in the inner aspect of upper and lower lids leading from the puncta to the common canaliculus and then to the tear sac.

Canthus: The angle at either end of the eyelid aperture—specified as inner or outer.

Cataract: Lens opacity.

Cataract extraction: Removal of a cataract by one of several methods.

Chalazion: Inflammation of a meibomian gland.

Chemosis: Conjunctival edema.

Choroid: Vascular middle coat between the retina and sclera.

Ciliary body: Portion of the uveal tract between the iris and the choroid including the ciliary processes and the ciliary muscle.

Coloboma: Congenital cleft due to the failure of some portion of the eye or ocular adnexa to complete growth.

Color blindness: Diminished ability to perceive differences in color.

Concave lens: Lens having the power to diverge rays of light. It is also known as negative, myopic, or minus lens, denoted by the sign (−).

Cones and rods: Two kinds of retinal receptor cells. Cones are concerned with visual acuity and color vision; rods, with peripheral vision under dim illumination.

Conjunctiva: Mucous membrane that lines the posterior aspect of the eyelids and the anterior sclera.

Convergence: The process of directing the visual axes of the eyes to a near point.

Convex lens: Lens having power to converge rays of light and to bring them into focus; also known as magnifying, hyperopic, or plus lens, denoted by the sign (+).

Cornea: Transparent portion of the outer coat of the eyeball forming the anterior wall of the aqueous chamber.

Corneal contact lenses: Thin lenses that fit directly on the cornea under the eyelids.

Corneal graft (keratoplasty): Surgery to restore vision by replacing a section of opaque cornea, either involving the full thickness of the cornea (penetrating keratoplasty) or only a superficial layer (lamellar keratoplasty).

Crystalline lens (or just the lens): A semi-transparent biconvex structure suspended in the eyeball between the aqueous and the vitreous. Its function is to bring rays of light to a focus on the retina.

Cycloplegic: A drug that temporarily relaxes the ciliary muscle, paralyzing accommodation.

Cylindrical lens: A segment of a cylinder, the refractive power of which varies in different meridians.

Dacryocystitis: Infection of the lacrimal sac.

Dark adaptation: The eyes' ability to adjust to decreased illumination.

Diopter: Unit of measurement that refers to the strength of refractive power in lenses or prisms.

Diplopia: Seeing one object as two.

"E" test: A system of testing visual acuity in illiterates, particularly preschool children.

Drusen: Small round yellow spots in or around the macula just outside the pigment epithelium. When in the optic nerve head, drusen appear as bumpy excrescences, which should not be confused with papilledema.

Dry-eye syndrome: Irritation secondary to decreased tearing.

Ectropion: Turning out of the eyelid.

Emmetropia: Absence of refractive error.

Endophthalmitis: Severe intraocular infection or inflammation.

Enophthalmos: Abnormal retro-displacement of the eyeball.

Entropion: A turning inward of the eyelid.

Enucleation: Complete surgical removal of the eyeball.

Episcleritis: Benign inflammation of the tissue between the conjunctiva and sclera.

Epiphora: Tearing.

Esophoria: A tendency of the eyes to turn inward.

Esotropia: A manifest inward deviation of the eyes.

Evisceration: Removal of the contents of the eyeball.

Exenteration: Removal of the entire contents of the orbit, including the eyeball and lids.

Exophoria: A tendency of the eyes to turn outward.

Exophthalmos: Abnormal protrusion of the eyeball.

Exotropia: A manifest outward deviation of one or both eyes.

Farsightedness: See Hyperopia.

Field of vision: the entire area that can be seen without shifting the gaze.

Floaters: Small dark particles in the vitreous.

Focus: The point to which rays are converged after passing through a lens. Focal distance is the distance between the lens and the focal point.

Fornix: The junction of the palpebral and bulbar conjunctiva.

Fovea: The center of the macula adapted for the most acute vision.

Fundus: The posterior portion of the eye, visible through an ophthalmoscope.

Fusion: Coordinating the images received by the two eyes into one image.

Glaucoma: Disease usually caused by elevated intraocular pressure, resulting in optic atrophy and loss of visual field.

Gonioscopy: A technique of examining the anterior angle, using a special corneal contact lens.

Hemianopia: Blindness of one half the field of vision in one or both eyes.

Hordeolum, external (sty): Infection of a hair follicle.

Hordeolum, internal: Infection of the meibomian gland.

Hyperopia, hypermetropia (farsightedness): A refractive error in which the focal point of light rays from a distant object is behind the retina.

Hyperphoria: A tendency of the eyes to deviate upward.

Hypertropia: A misalignment of the eyes whereby the visual axis of one eye is higher than the fellow fixating eye.

Hyphema: Blood in the anterior chamber.

Hypopyon: Pus in the anterior chamber.

Hypotony: Abnormally soft eye from any cause.

Injection: Congestion of blood vessels.

Iris: Circular membrane (the color part, e.g., brown, blue, green) suspended behind the cornea and in front of the lens.

Jaeger test: A test for near vision using lines of various sizes of type.

Keratoconus: Cone-shaped deformity of the cornea.

Keratomalacia: Softening of the cornea, usually associated with vitamin A deficiency.

Keratoplasty: Cornea transplant (graft).

Lacrimal sac: The dilated area at the junction of the nasolacrimal duct and the canaliculi.

Lesion: Injury.

Lens (Crystalline lens): A refractive medium having one or both curved surfaces.

Leukoma: Dense corneal opacity due to any cause.

Limbus: Junction of the cornea and sclera.

Macula lutea (or just macula): (Latin: macula=spot; lutea=yellow). The round or somewhat oval avascular center of the retina used for central vision.

Metamorphopsia: Wavy distortion of vision.

Microphthalmos: Abnormal smallness of the eyeball.

Miotic: A drug causing pupillary constriction.

Mydriatic: A drug causing pupillary dilatation.

Myokymia: Twitching of eyelids, usually a benign transient condition, probably related to fatigue or tension. It is usually unilateral.

Myopia (nearsightedness): A refractive error in which the focal point for light rays from a distant object is anterior to the retina.

Neovascularization: Formation of new blood vessels.

Nicking (arteriovenous or AV nicking): a phenomenon whereby a small artery crosses a small vein, resulting in bulging on either side of the intersection.

Nystagmus: An involuntary, rapid movement of the eyeball that may be horizontal, vertical, rotatory, or mixed.

Oculist: An outdated term for ophthalmologist, a physician who is a specialist in diseases of the eye.

Ophthalmic neonatorum: Conjunctivitis in a newborn.

Ophthalmoscope: An instrument with a special illumination system for viewing the inside of the eye, particularly the retina and associated structures.

Optic atrophy: Optic nerve degeneration.

Optic disc: The visible portion of the optic nerve inside the eye.

Optic nerve: The nerve that carries visual impulses from the retina to the brain.

Optician: A person who makes or deals in glasses or other optical instruments and who fills prescriptions for glasses.

Optometrist: A non-physician trained in the examination and measurement of refraction of the eye. In some states they are licensed to treat some eye conditions.

Orthoptist: A person who gives training to those with ocular muscle imbalances.

Palpebral: Pertaining to the eyelid.

Pannus: Infiltration of the cornea with blood vessels.

Papilledema: Swelling of the optic disc.

Perimeter: An instrument for measuring the field of vision.

Peripheral vision: Ability to perceive the presence, motion, or color of objects outside the direct line of vision.

Photocoagulation: A method, usually involving a laser, to artificially burn the retina and choroid for treatment of certain types of retinal disorders such as diabetic retinopathy or retinal detachment.

Photophobia: Abnormal sensitivity to light.

Photopsia: Appearance of flashes or sparks within the eye due to irritation of the retina, usually caused by the vitreous pulling on it.

Phthisis bulbi: Atrophy of the eyeball with blindness and decreased intraocular pressure, due to end-stage intraocular disease.

Pinguecula: A benign, usually yellowish, soft, slightly elevated area found typically nasal to the cornea, less often lateral.

Posterior chamber: Space filled with aqueous, anterior to the lens and posterior to the iris.

Presbyopia: Blurred near vision (old sight) usually evident after age 40, due to reduction in the ability of the lens to accommodate.

Pseudophakia: Presence of an artificial intraocular lens implant following cataract extraction.

Pterygium: A growth of tissue (usually triangular) that extends from the conjunctiva over the cornea.

Ptosis: Drooping of the eyelid.

Puncta: External orifices of the upper and lower canaliculi.

Pupil: The round hole in the center of the iris.

Refraction: In relation to ophthalmology, the determination of refractive errors of the eye and correction by glasses. In physics, the deviation in the course of rays of light in passing from one transparent medium into another of different density.

Refractive error: A defect that prevents light rays from being brought to a single focus on the retina.

Refractive media: The transparent parts of the eye having refractive power.

Retina: The innermost layer of the eye, consisting of the sensory retina, which is composed of light-sensitive neural elements connecting to other neural cells, and the pigment epithelium.

Retinal detachment: A separation of the retina from the choroid.

Retinitis pigmentosa: A hereditary degeneration and atrophy of the retina.

Retinoblastoma: A rare malignant retinal tumor that affects young children.

Retinoscope: An instrument for testing the objective aspect of refraction.

Rods: Retinal receptor cells concerned with peripheral vision under decreased illumination.

Rubeosis: Growth of abnormal vessels on the iris, signifying ischemia of the retina.

Sclera: The tough white covering of the eye that, along with the cornea, forms the external protective coat of the eye.

Scotoma: A blind or partially blind area in the visual field.

Slit lamp: A microscope with a special light source for examination of the eye, principally the anterior segment.

Snellen chart: A chart drawn to Snellen measurement, consisting of letters or numbers in graded sizes for testing central visual acuity.

Strabismus (heterotropia): A manifest deviation of the eyes.

Sty (External hordeolum): Infection of a hair follicle along the lid.

Sympathetic ophthalmia: Inflammation in one eye following injury (traumatic inflammation) in the fellow eye.

Synechia: Adhesion of the iris to the cornea (anterior synechia) or lens (posterior synechia).

Syneresis: A degenerative process within the vitreous gel.

Telangiectasia: An area with excessive numbers of small blood vessels.

Tonometer: An instrument for measuring intraocular pressure.

Trachoma: A serious infection of the conjunctiva and cornea caused by a chlamydial infection.

Trichiasis: Inward turning of eyelashes against the eye, resulting in ocular irritation and sometimes damage.

Tropia: Strabismus.

Uvea (uveal tract): The iris, ciliary body and choroid.

Uveitis: Inflammation of one or all portions of the uveal tract.

Visual acuity: Detailed central vision.

Vitreous: Transparent, colorless gel filling the eyeball behind the lens.

Zonule: The fine tissue strands that stretch from the ciliary processes to the lens equator (360 degrees) and hold the lens in place.

Made in the USA
Thornton, CO
04/26/22 14:48:03

9738a516-7630-4d9a-be40-52ba036678faR02